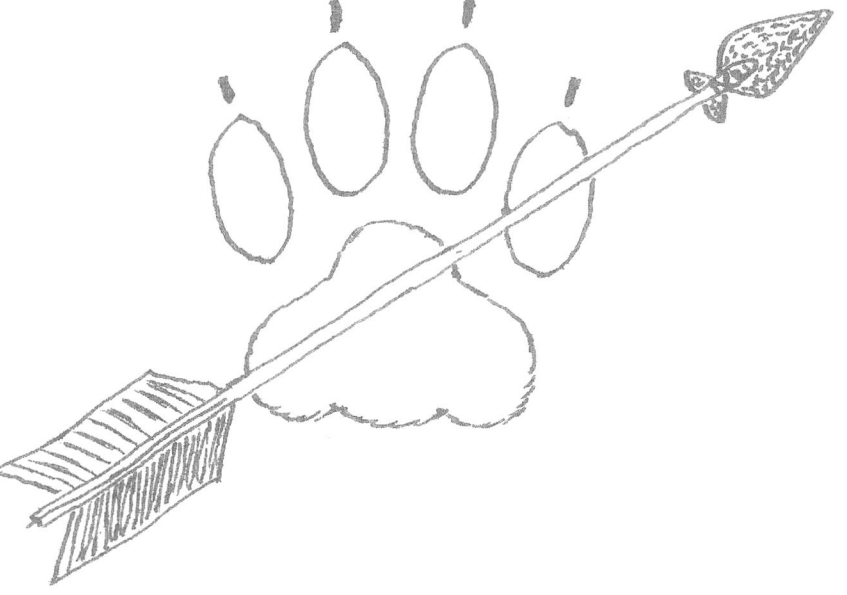

Cover photo: The author meditates before an afternoon full of blindfolded training. Equal parts Dread Pirate Roberts, Zatoichi, and Kenobi style training.

Share the Gift

FROM THE TRAINING
JOURNALS OF
AARON F. DILL

Share the Gift
From the Training Journals of Aaron F Dill
Copyright ©2020 by Aaron F Dill

All rights reserved. No portion of this book may be reproduced or transmitted in any form or by any means without written permission from the author

ISBN 9798657295122

The exercises, ideas, and suggestions in this book are not intended as a substitute for professional medical advice. Always consult a physician or healthcare professional before beginning any new exercise technique or exercise program, or if you are elderly, or if you have any recurring medical or psychological conditions. Any application of the exercises, ideas, and suggestions in this book is at the reader's sole discretion and risk.

The author and publisher of this book and their employers and employees make no warranty of any kind regarding the content of this book including, but not limited to, any implied warranties of merchantability, or fitness for any purpose. The author and publisher of this book and their employers and employees are not liable or responsible to any person or entity for any errors contained in this document, or for any special, incidental, or consequential damage caused or alleged to be caused directly or indirectly by the information contained in this book.

Risks involved in the practices detailed in this book include, but are by no means limited to, improved health, greater strength, deeper enjoyment of life, even better looks, and higher levels of charm.

Introduction

I've kept training journals for years illustrating with diagrams specific to the notes or just with sketches and art that catches my attention. Once in a while I would share excerpts of particularly good pages. A few friends asked me to share more of my notes, but I wasn't ready, and I didn't really envision ever sharing a lot. But the seed was planted, and I wondered if my journals could become something.

I let one good friend read the whole thing and she said "you could publish this!" but I felt the format was too raw and unorganized. But that seed started to stir and send out roots.

A couple friends from Toronto visited our farm last summer and when I brought out my training journal to jot down some of the herbs and book titles we were talking about they said "Oh, the infamous notebook!" It hit me that it was time to shape the raw collection into a cohesive, artistic resource worthy of sharing. And so the seed grew and sent up shoots.

I ran the idea by a brother, and he encouraged me strongly. So I began to draft and write. And the shoots put on leaves.

The fruit of my effort is now in your hands.

Acknowledgements

Thanks to many people in my life and throughout history, who have shared their gifts through teaching and writing.

Special thanks to two masters and living legends from whom I have had the privilege to learn in person - Tom Brown Jr of Tracker School and Vladimir Vasiliev of Systema HQ.

Thanks to my Systema and Tracker families around the globe: training with you and learning from you are many of my favorite memories.

Thanks to my Senseis and friends at the Emmett Judo Club and the Western Idaho Judo Institute who so selflessly share their love of Judo.

Thanks to my Idaho brotherband: Josiah, Jesse, and Jacob. Whether we're climbing mountains, throwing each other on the mats, or just enjoying a beer and a campfire, I'm thankful for your fellowship and the good times.

Thanks to my family for supporting this project and for hours of proofreading.

Heather, thank you. I love bouncing ideas with you and swinging kettlebells together. I love you.

Thanks to Kerry McQuisten for her generous advice on navigating the self-publishing process; and Michael Beal for his computer skills and formatting.

And thanks to you, who took the jump to buy a new book from a first time author. I hope you enjoy it and find something helpful for your journey.

"To whom much has been given, much will be required."
I have been given much; and I will share what I have learned. Take this and pass it on. Share the gift.

All the best,
Aaron
11. Aug. 2020

SDG

Contents

Part 1: Strength
Quotes
Breathwork
Systema Core 4
Quotes
Breath for Internal Control
Moving on the ground
Convict Conditioning
Kettlebell: Simple & Sinister
The Quick and the Dead
Hillsprints
Havadlos
Mornat
Train Outside
Training Log
Exercises
Quotes

Part 2: Health
Daily Maintainance
Injury Protocol
Tension Waves for Deeper Relaxation
Breath for Healing
Enter the Douse

Vitamin D
Massage
Apple Cider Vinegar
Water
Fasting
Foraging
Maffetone Method
Diet or No-diet
Organic
Grass fed & grass finished
Healthy Fat!
Pat Moe - Diet Advice
Quotes

Part 3: Further Training and Thoughts
Quotes
Every Day Carry
Vehicle Kit
Preparedness
100 Skills Every Man Should Know
Why do we do what we do?
Quotes
Awareness
Awareness Test from Tom Brown, Jr.
Sit Spot
Survival Awareness Tracker School notes

Fox Walk
Tracker School Stories
The Fox and the Skunk
Quotes
Systema
Judo Notes
Judo Notes: Tank vs. Sniper
The Growth Mindset
Archery
Gunfighters Prayer
Tribe
Practice List 2015
Quotes
Deeper Preparedness and Local Reliance
Blindwork
Short Swords
Physical Training is a Bare Minimum
Keep Fear to Yourself, Share Courage with Others
Books
Quotes
The Prayer of the Optina Elders
Peace is elusive
Final Quotes

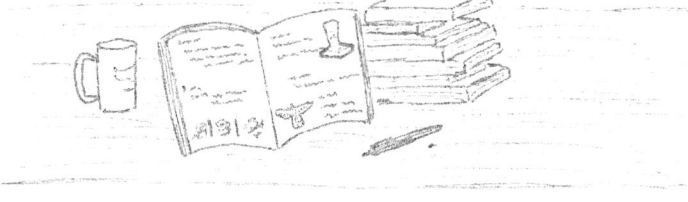

Part 1: Strength

No citizen has the right
to be an amateur in the
matter of physical training.
What a disgrace it is
for a man to grow old
without ever seeing the
beauty and strength of
which his body is capable.
— Socrates

People will look and know,
"These people are ready
to fight the dragons at the
gate. They long to slaughter
dragons."
They will know this,
because they have witnessed
you training to fight dragons
— mountain guerilla
"Forging the Hero"

A workout should be a short, sharp session that leaves you feeling recharged, energized, and invigorated. Not a long, drawn-out affair that grinds you down and leaves you sore and aching for days.

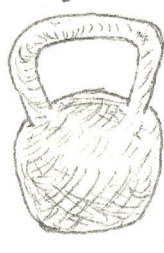

"MORE IS NOT BETTER, IT'S JUST MORE."
— Steve Baccari

Always leave some gas in the tank. I want to be ready to go at a moment's notice to defend myself or save a life, or if the neighborhood kids want to play, or if a buddy calls for help moving a fridge, or if my cows get out.

Moderate daily training
is the ticket to being
always ready.
The purpose of a training
session is to store
energy in the body,
not exhaust it.
— Pavel, Strongfirst

Natural movements
heal us.
And if they are new,
they develop
us too.
— Vladimir Vasiliev

The perfect blend of
sophistication and
savagery.
— Savage Gentleman

Breathwork

We use breathwork - slow calisthenics and natural movements connected to breathing patterns and breath holds - to strengthen body, mind, and spirit to function calmly and efficiently under stress, and to absorb or deflect the various impacts of life, without damage to ourselves.

Slow calisthenics emphasize tendon strength and joint health, and connecting breathing to movement increases oxygenation of the blood for physical capacity and mental clarity.

> Awareness without breathing is only half the control.
> — Vladimir Vasiliev

START INHALE — START MOVE — FINISH MOVE — FINISH INHALE   same with exhale

Breath should encompass every move. Lead with your breath.

Since oxygen is one of our most basic needs, holding the breath is one of the fastest ways to induce a helpful level of panic response for training purposes. It brings up tensions and fears, and then by breathing again you can relax them.

Breath holds also train our stress response to be automatically starting to breathe more, whether we are nervous, afraid, or in pain.

Burst breathing:

Use burst breathing to recover from breath holds or strenuous exertion. Light fast breathing, in through the nose out through the mouth. Do not breathe so deep that you create more tension, but rather 'bounce' your breath off the tension and then breathe deeper as your tension relaxes and recedes.

Systema Core 4

Push ups: hands directly beneath your shoulders, either palms or fists are fine. Keep elbows close to your body, flaring elbows wide can be rough on your shoulders. Keep body straight like a plank, don't dip head or bend at the waist.
Push ups from your knees are perfectly acceptable if thats what your strength allows.

Squats: feet shoulder-width apart. Try to point feet straight forward, but they can point out a little if your hips are tight.
Keep your feet flat on the ground, heels down.
Knees track in line with toes, but don't go forward past your toes.
Keep your back straight, not necessarily vertical, but straight.
Don't slump. Keep your head up and look around.
If your knees grind or pop try to focus on pushing the earth away instead of muscling yourself up.

Sit ups: from laying down, bend at the waist to sit up.
Arms stay relaxed at your sides, definitely don't pull yourself up.
Leave your legs flat on the ground, if your feet want to rise as you sit up, relax your hips.
Keep your back as straight as possible.

Leg raises: from laying down, raise legs up to 90° or all the way over your head to touch the ground behind you.
Legs stay straight
Press lower back into the ground, until feet are past 90°.
Exhale as you raise legs and compress diaphragm, inhale as you lower legs and expand.

- Start with 5/5/5/5 or 10/10/10/10 to limber up, or repeat in a series.
- Connect an inhale or exhale to each rise or lower.

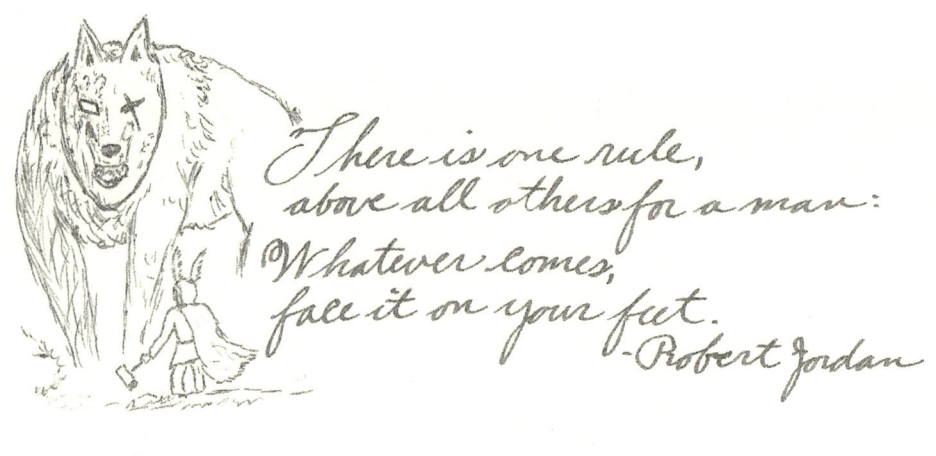

There is one rule, above all others for a man: Whatever comes, face it on your feet.
— Robert Jordan

"We must be masters of adaptability in a world of ambiguity."
— Pat McNamara

"The art of living is more like wrestling than dancing, because an artful life requires being prepared to meet and withstand sudden and unexpected attacks."
— Marcus Aurelius

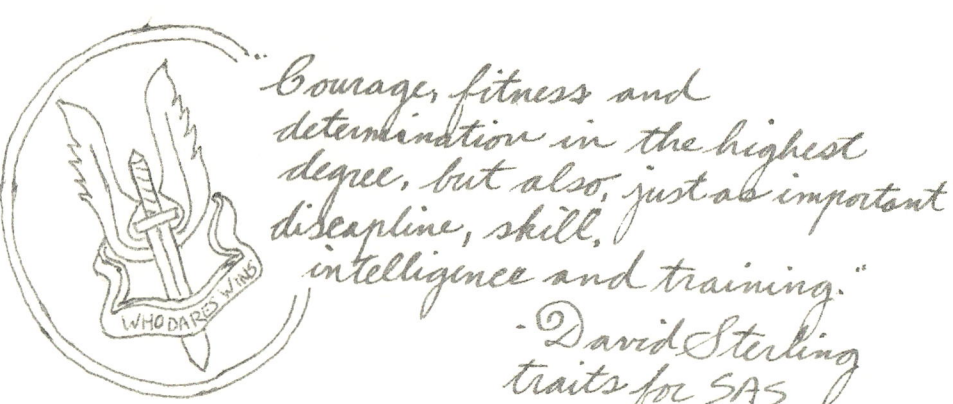

"Courage, fitness and determination in the highest degree, but also, just as important discipline, skill, intelligence and training."
— David Sterling
traits for SAS

Breath for Internal Control
Vladimir Vasiliev
Systema HQ

- Sit or lay down and pause for a minute to take note of your state of relaxation.

- Get into push up position, exhale, hold your breath, do one push up. Breathe to recover and sit until you are as relaxed as when you started, or more so.
Repeat with two, three, four, etc.
Keep your pace even.

- Same for squats, sit ups, and leg raises.

> Tens are easily attainable twenties are a good goal. Vlad said Russian operators would work up to forties.

- Walk, hold your breath on exhale count your steps. When can't hold any longer, run and breathe to recover. Then repeat. If you recover correctly, you will hold your breath further each time.

Moving on the ground

Strength begins with movement.
You must be able to move freely
before you can move strongly.

※

Moving on the ground is a fantastic
warm up as well as a mobility check.
It also acts as a form of massage;
anything tight or tense tends to stick
out and get massaged by the floor.

※

Start by laying on your back;
   roll onto your stomach, then roll back.
          Easy.

※

Boring? wait a minute.
Lead the roll with your hand or foot,
imagine you are pushing something
further and further until your body
follows and rolls over.
Or, imagine a line tied to your
wrist or ankle, pulling you to
   roll over.

Or put your arms and legs in the air and move forward, backward, and sideways by inching your spine (great for your back!).

※

Or sit up (try without muscles — that will keep your brain busy for a minute), and then fall back down in any direction. You can come up to your knees or even standing and then go back down.

※

Add in shoulder rolls and back rolls, or a back roll into a handstand if you are ambitious.

※

Get the point? The opportunities and varieties are almost endless. Strive to keep your movement smooth and relaxed and free.

Explore. Enjoy.

※

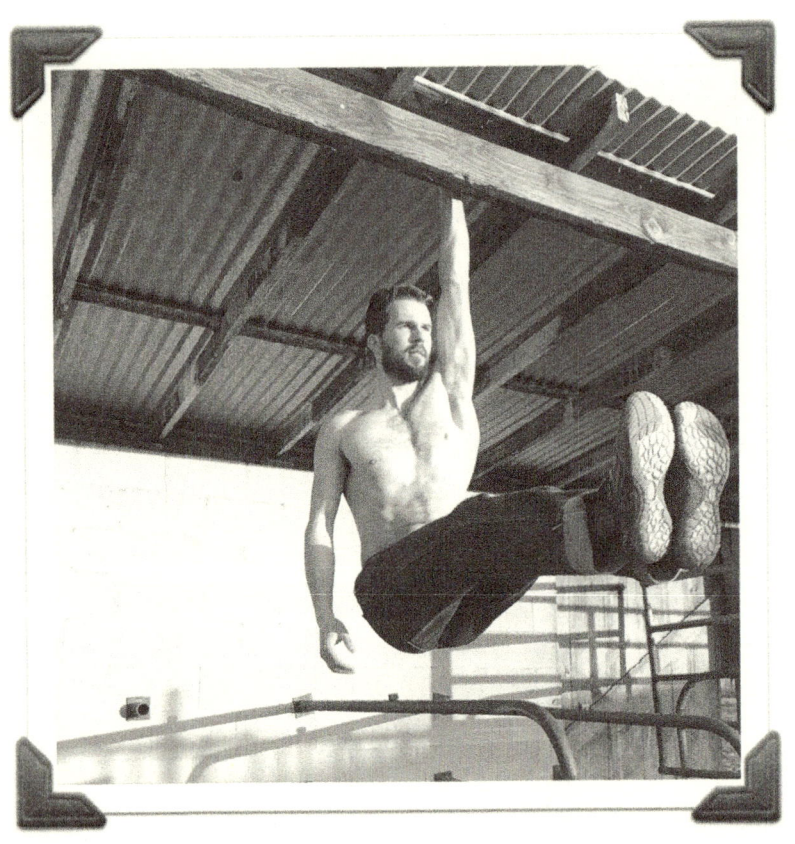

Most physical training systems are designed for the domesticated human animal. That is to say, for us humans who live lives of such relative security that we cultivate our strength and power more out of pride and for a sense of accomplishment than out of an absolute need to survive in the wild.
The professional athlete hones his body to function well in a sports event — rather than to emerge safe from a life-or-death struggle.
— Convict Conditioning

Convict Conditioning by Paul Wade

Convict Conditioning is a brilliant system utilizing progressive calisthenics. The Big Six - pull ups, push ups, squats, legraises, bridges, and handstands - are broken down into 10 step series from a basic version that anyone can do, up to elite versions like one-arm push ups or pistol squats.

IT'S DEFINITELY WRITTEN TOWARD A MASCULINE AUDIENCE, BUT THE INFO IS GOOD FOR EVERYONE.

Convict Conditioning 2 deals with the "shotgun muscles" - grip, neck, calves, and the lateral chain; as well as active stretching (Trifecta: L-sit, bridge, and seated twist holds), and the importance of regular meals and plenty of sleep.

PULL-UPS
SQUATS
GRIP
PUSH-UPS
LEG RAISES
CALVES
HANDSTANDS
BRIDGES
NECK

M: PULL-UPS + GRIP
T: BRIDGES + NECK
OR W: HANDSTAND
Th: LEGRAISES + FLAG
F: SQUATS + CALVES
S: PUSH-UPS
Su: REST
OR MIX IT UP HOWEVER YOU LIKE.

LIMIT YOUR SETS, BUT PUSH YOUR REPS ALMOST TO FAILURE, WITHOUT LOSING FORM. KEEP THEM CLEAN!

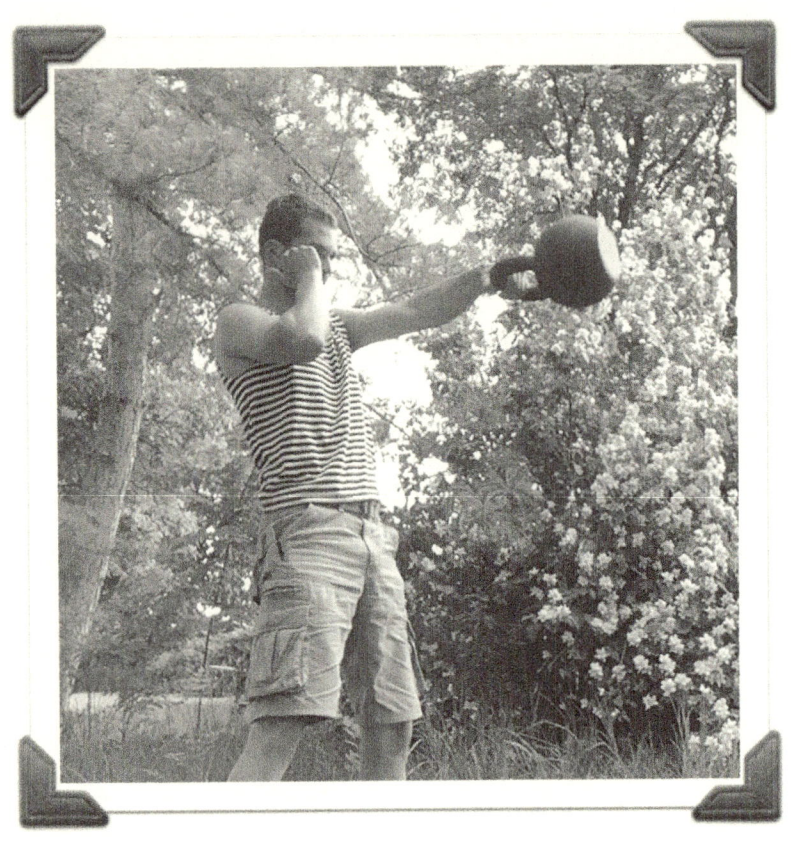

I used to be a calisthenics-only guy. Simple & Sinister changed that. Kettlebell up!

Kettlebell: Simple & Sinister
Pavel, Strongfirst

My favorite kettlebell plan; straight-forward and to the point.

- warm up - 3 circuits of 5 each: prying goblet squats, shoulder bridges, and kettlebell halos (both directions)

- recharge session: 10 x 10 swings
  5 x 1 get-ups (per side)

Scalable to many ability levels, start with a comfortable weight and as Pavel says, "repeat until strong."

DO SWINGS FASTER THAN COMFORTABLE, GET-UPS SLOWER THAN COMFORTABLE.
    - PAVEL

GUYS: START WITH 16KG & 24KG.
GIRLS: START WITH 8KG & 12KG
OR A 5KG ROCK FOR GET-UPS

The 'Talk Test': rest between sets should be just long enough that your breathing and heartrate slow to where you can form a complete sentence. Then get back to it!

Own the bell. Don't _ever_ sacrifice form.

StrongFirst Q&D, my other favorite kettlebell program.

I did this 3x a week for two months, and while my numbers on the scale didn't change, a friend who has done bodywork for us for years said my muscle felt more dense; it wasn't tension, just heavy.

I trained M, W, F before breakfast for optimal health and endurance.

The science behind this program is fascinating! Timing and explosive power are crucial for stimulating and training the mitochondrial powerhouse.

> LEAVE METCONS, EXHAUSTION, STIFFNESS, AND SORENESS TO PREY. STAY FRESH TO HUNT ANOTHER DAY.
> — PAVEL in Q&D

GET THE BOOK AND READ ABOUT IT!

Bear in mind, this is an advanced program. Beginners are better served by S&S or a steady calisthenic program.

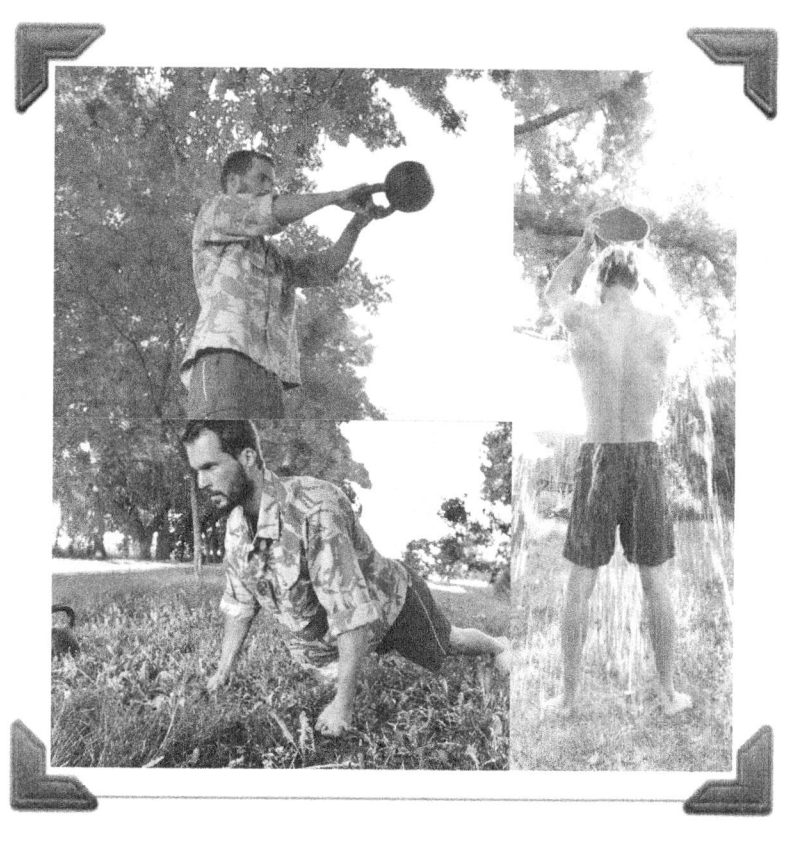

Q & D plus a cold douse, a great way to start the day.

A view from a get-up.

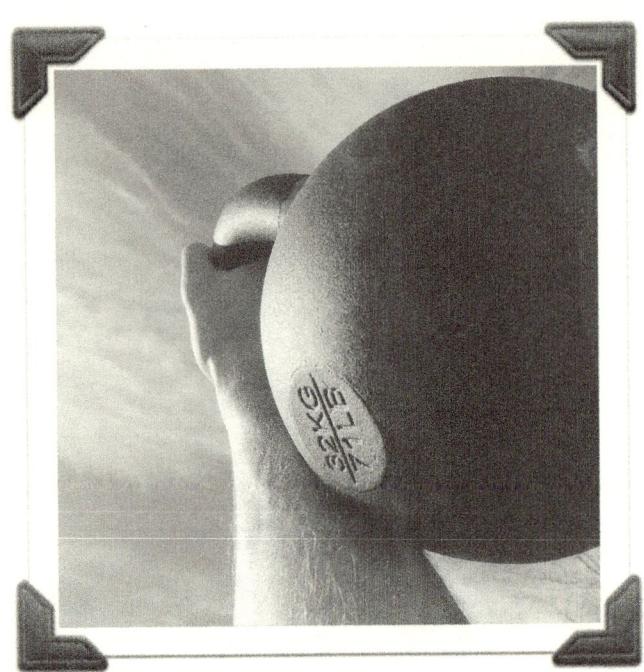

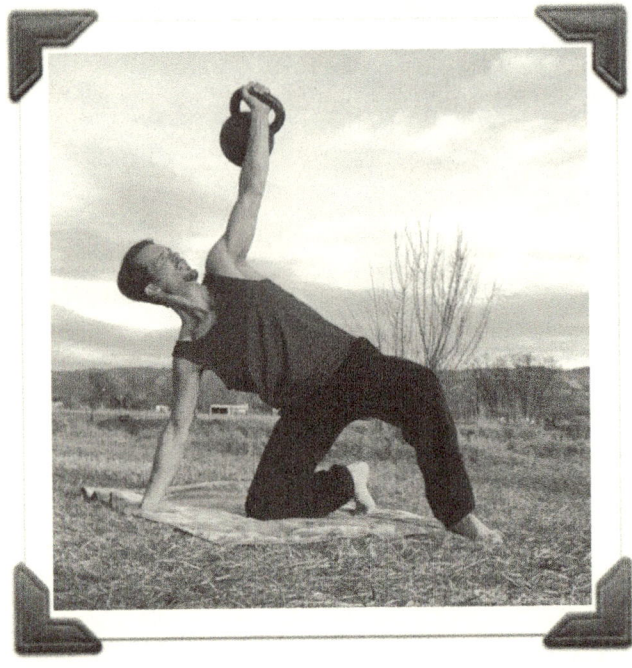

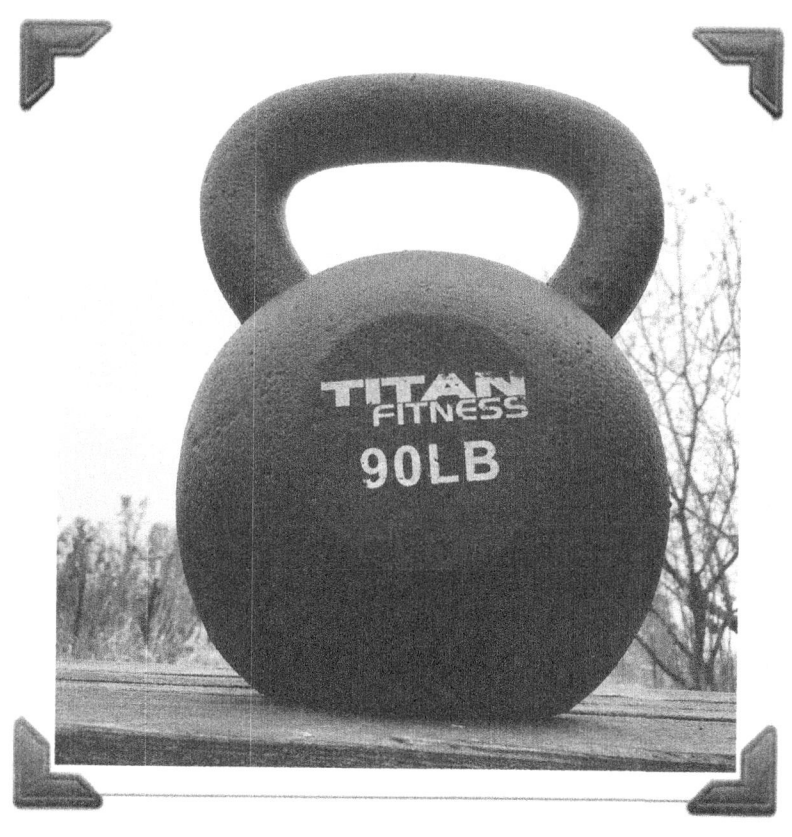

Dec. 2019. Bought a new paperweight

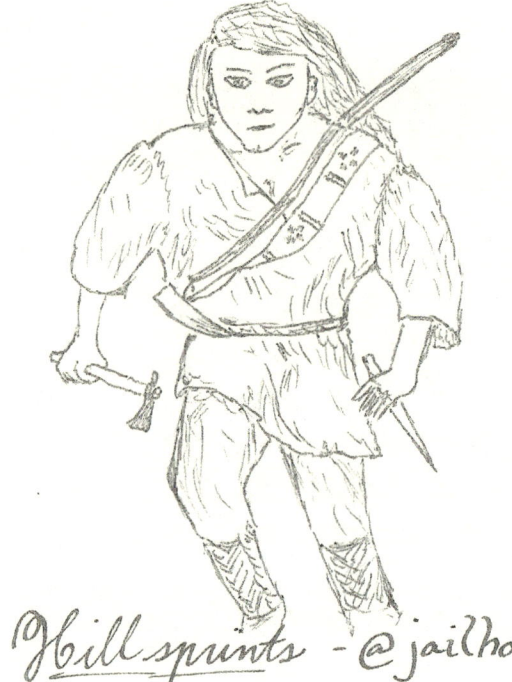

Hill sprints - @jailhousestrong

Hill sprints unlock something
that neither the weight room
or the track can access.
Hill sprints are very intense
but relatively safe, and catalyze
power production, speed, fat burning,
and mental toughness in record time.

Find a hill and run it!
Or a set of stairs, those are good, too.

Kavadlo Bros

Al and Danny Kavadlo are tattooed humorous masters of calisthenics, with a gift for teaching and encouraging.

"HEY
 HEY
  HEY!

WE'RE
WORKING
OUT!"

I've read "Raising the Bar," "Everybody needs Training" and "Get Strong." And I would recommend anything with their name on it!

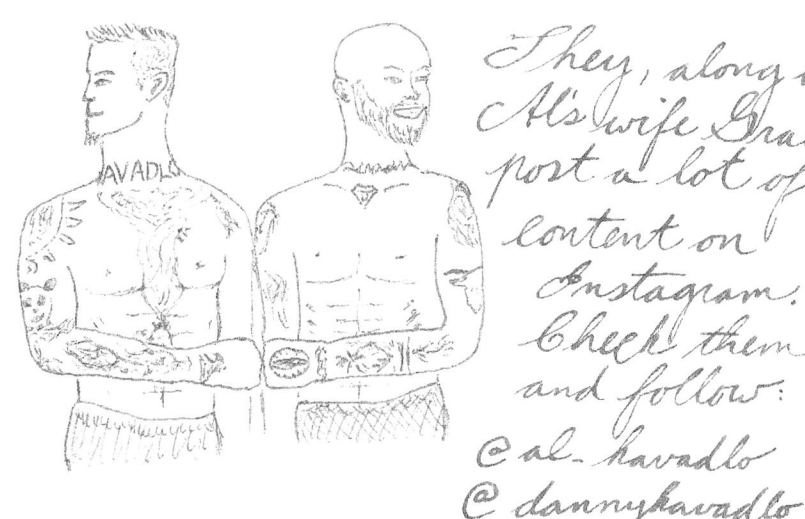

They, along with Al's wife Grace, post a lot of good content on Instagram. Check them out and follow:

@al_kavadlo
@dannykavadlo
@grace_kavadlo

MOUNAT

Erwin Le Corre's system of natural movement. Watch his video "The Workout the World Forgot"; he's barefoot and clad in running shorts, charging through jungle and up hills, running along the guard wall of a bridge, climbing trees, scaling boulders, carrying large rocks and logs, swimming up a clear river, and diving deep into the ocean.

Exploring his capabilities, and expanding his limits.

You can too.

Start with simple stuff. Walk barefoot outside. Sit down on the ground. Climb a tree. Pick up a rock or other moderately heavy but asymetric object. Go for a light jog. Crawl on all fours. Enjoy!

10 Aspects of natural movement

- **Pursuit** — walk
  - run
  - crawl
- **Escape** — climb
  - balance
  - jump
  - swim
- **Attack** — throw
  - lift
  - fight

> "EVERY CHILD SHOULD LEARN TO SWIM, RIDE AND FIGHT."
> — HELIO GRACIE

> "BE STRONG TO BE USEFUL."
> — GEORGES HÉBERT

> "When children play, they're really role-playing disasters. Turn them loose and they'll run, wrestle, hide, roll around, kick-fight with their feet, and leap off anything they can climb — exactly the skills that could keep them alive in a real emergency."
> — Christopher McDougal, 'Natural Born Heroes'

I train outside as much as I can. Fresh free air, sunshine, and quiet solitude; recharge for body, mind, and soul.

I HAVE A BARN WITH A SOUTH FACE THAT MAKES A GOOD SOLAR REFLECTOR AND WIND BREAK FOR COLD MONTHS, & SHADE TREES CLOSE BY FOR SUMMER TIME.

Tom Brown said Grandfather always insisted they workout outside, so they would be used to working hard in all conditions, not just pleasant days or controlled climates.

You don't need a lot of space or equipment, just enough room to move a bit.

Pavel talks about a "courage corner" - just a designated area with a few kettlebells and a pull up bar. Apparently these are common in Russian military bases and even submarines, and soldiers will drop in during the course of the day to put in a 20 to 40 min session before continuing on with their duties.

Training log: I find journaling or writing down workouts to be quite a helpful tool.

I like being able to go back and see exactly what I was doing six months or a year ago. Seeing the improvements march along through the pages is encouraging when you put in steady work; or if you take a couple days off, it's a hard record of exactly how long.

It's also useful in the event of an injury to look at where overtraining/under-recovery contributed.

Just get a cheap notebook and jot down a line or two.

SUCH AS:

15. May. 19
2x 1 min handstand
5+1 each side pistol squats

4. July. 19
Murph - 20 lb vest, calisthenics unweighted. 56 min.

13. Nov. 19
S&S - swings: 1 hand 32 kg
get ups: 32 kg

There are two types of people who focus on their fundamentals:

The very new, and the very advanced.

DON'T GLORIFY COMPLICATION. SIMPLE IS GOLD.

~~~~~~~~~~~~~~~~~~~

Get-ups: shift your hips an inch or two toward your loaded side, this makes the first stage much easier. Also focus on grip, crush the bell; put your power up into your hand.

Dead-hang: grab a pull-up bar and just hang. Good for grip and core.

Bear crawls: forward, backward, side-to-side. Works coordination, upper body and general conditioning. Great grapplers exercise. If, God forbid, you're ever under fire you better know how to get low and move fast. Besides, there is something primal in quadripedal movement.

Kettlebell swings: power from the hips do the Russian style, up to chin or chest height, but not higher for shoulder injury.

Pull ups: a favorite of mine since I started Boy Scouts at 13. Back when they still required pull ups.

Bottoms-up press: balance a light kettlebell upside down and press it up. Maintain balance! Fantastic for stabilizers in shoulders and core and heals shoulder injury.
I used bottoms-up presses with 16 kg to train for a 32 kg clean and press (kettlebell).

Pistol squats: practice in a doorway for balance if you need, or grab your non-working foot with same-side hand. Bodyweight or with a kettlebell.

Burpee & kettlebell snatches: brutal and efficient.

Muscle up: the king of calisthenics and bodyweight exercise.

Start by doing what
is necessary;
Then do what is possible;
And suddenly you are doing
the impossible.
— St. Francis of Assisi

Sometimes it's lack of patience
that leads to lack of progress.
Things take time.
We have to respect that...
— Emmanuel Manolakakis

GOOD THINGS TAKE TIME.

BEING STRONG IS A CHOICE. SO IS BEING WEAK.

You have power of your mind —
not outside events.
Realize this and you will
find strength.
— Marcus Aurelius

It is the love of life.
That is why we train so hard,
so you can preserve life.
— Guru Dan Inosanto

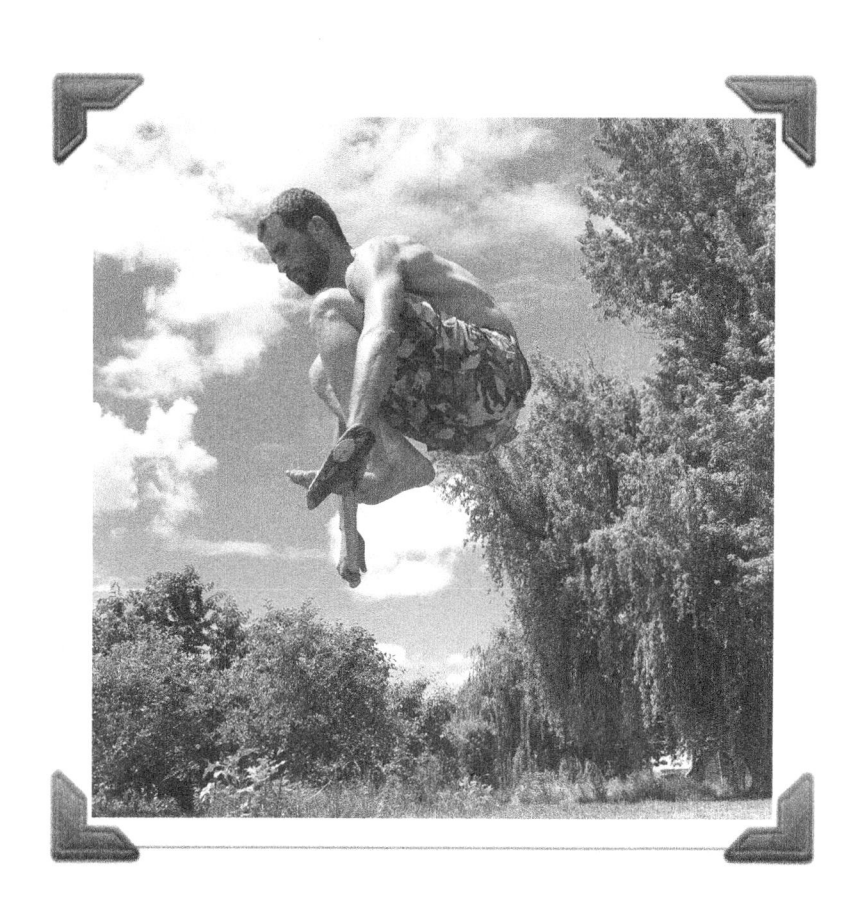

Movement is life, enjoy it!
Go have fun!

Part 2: Health

Daily Maintainance

- drink a quart of water within half an hour of waking up. Preferably with a teaspoon of ACV (apple cider vinegar)

- take a few minutes to roll out any stiffness with a PVC roller, soft ball, or joint circles

- golf ball your feet

- douse (at least 2 or 3 x week)

Injury Protocol

- self massage with roller, softball and roll a golfball under your feet
- get bodywork
- arnica: salve or gel, and homeopathic
  - 3 or 4x daily, or whenever sore
- check diaphragm tension
  - massage, breathing
- breathe through injured area
  - imagine air flowing directly in
- check emotional/spiritual baggage
  - what weight are you carrying?
- review recent movement patterns
  - are you over using / under recovering, or using poor mechanics?
- gentle stretching, then careful calisthenics
- cut back sugar, caffeine, alcohol, processed carbs
- focus on lots of water (with ACV), green tea, healthy fats, leafy greens, and berries.

I roll on a softball around my scapulas to iron out residues of old shoulder injuries.

I use a 3" x 3' schedule 40 PVC pipe to roll on up and down my back and neck and for large muscles.

And I have a golfball to roll under my feet to stimulate the lymphatic system and reflexology points that connect throughout the body. That gentle motion also felt really good on a sore knee.

SIMPLE TOOLS

Tension waves for <u>deeper relaxation</u>

Tense the body in a wave from feet up to head with an inhale, then relax in a wave from head down to feet with an exhale. You can reverse directions to tense from head down and relax feet up, or tense and relax in the same direction, or flip the breathing to tense on exhale and relax with inhale, or tensing the whole body all at once and relax all at once.

Also, tensing part of your body while keeping everything else relaxed: inhale, tense one arm; exhale, relax; inhale, tense both legs; exhale, relax; inhale, tense torso; exhale, relax; inhale, tense one arm and one leg; exhale, relax. etc.

Study how to tense one part rock hard while leaving everything else loose.

SOURCE: "LET EVERY BREATH..."
"THE RUSSIAN SYSTEM GUIDEBOOK"

Breath for healing

Breathe through various areas of your body, especially injuries. Imagine air flowing directly in through that area. You can do this in a wave through the whole body, or target specific areas.

Vlad said soldiers in his unit were taught to heal themselves this way. We can too.

You can do any of these exercises (tension waves or breathing) in a variety of positions; standing, walking, or laying down.

I often go through a few in the course of a day to check tension or help release it.

These are also really nice for helping go to sleep if you are restless, or gently waking up in the morning.

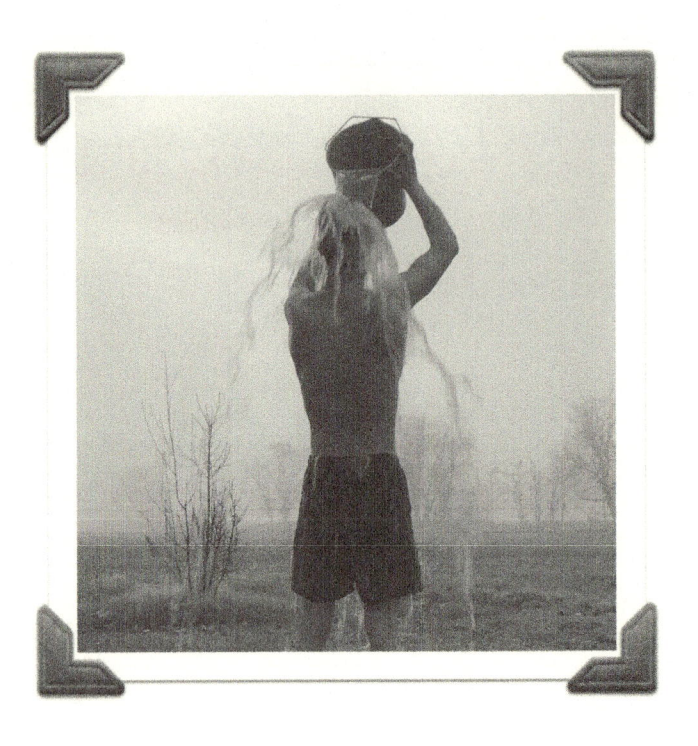

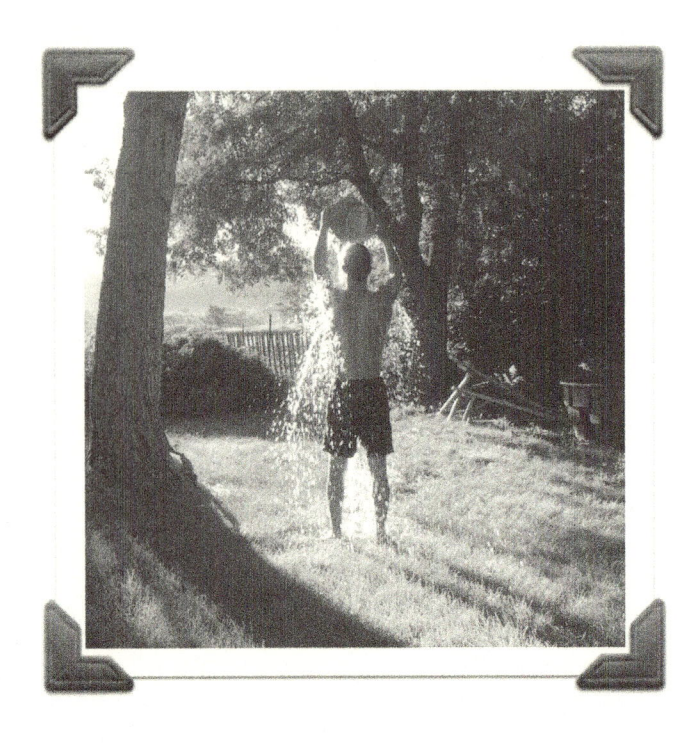

Enter the Douse

I picked up dousing from my friends at Systema HQ, and shortly after found Wim Hof's research.

> "THE COLD IS MERCILESS, BUT IT IS RIGHTEOUS."
> —WIM HOF

I douse regularly in all seasons, and have found it improved my cold tolerance and circulation significantly. Pouring a bucket of cold water over your head is a powerful practice. Cold is one of the fastest ways to fire up your metabolism, and to stimulate and strengthen your central nervous system and overall immune system.

It's also an exercise in will power; denying yourself small simple things —like a hot shower— go a surprisingly long way in building mental fortitude and resiliance.

Douse when your body is warm; it feels phenomenal after a workout or stretching session.

Or it's a great way to kickstart your day. Then drink some hot tea or coffee to help warm up again.

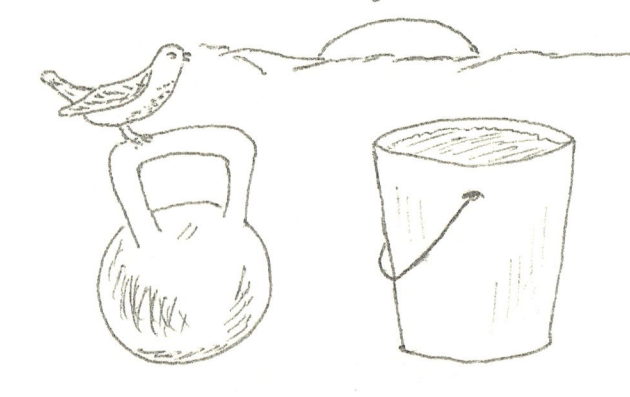

SUNRISE, BIRDSONG, AND COLD WATER CASCADING OVER MY HEAD.

Cold showers are good, too. My dad taught me to always finish a warm shower with a few seconds of cold to close the pores. Later I added completely cold showers; I don't always forego hot water, but it's an option.

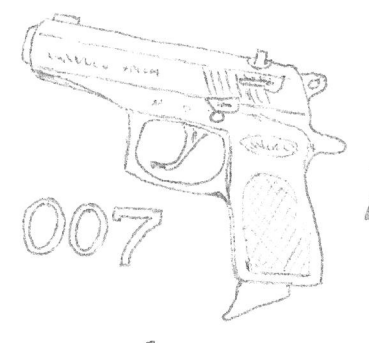

James Bond always finishes his showers cold, too.

It's unpleasant to contemplate stepping into a shower of cold water, invigorating to do so, and then after 20-30 seconds my body adjusts and it's quite enjoyable.

Embrace the cold!

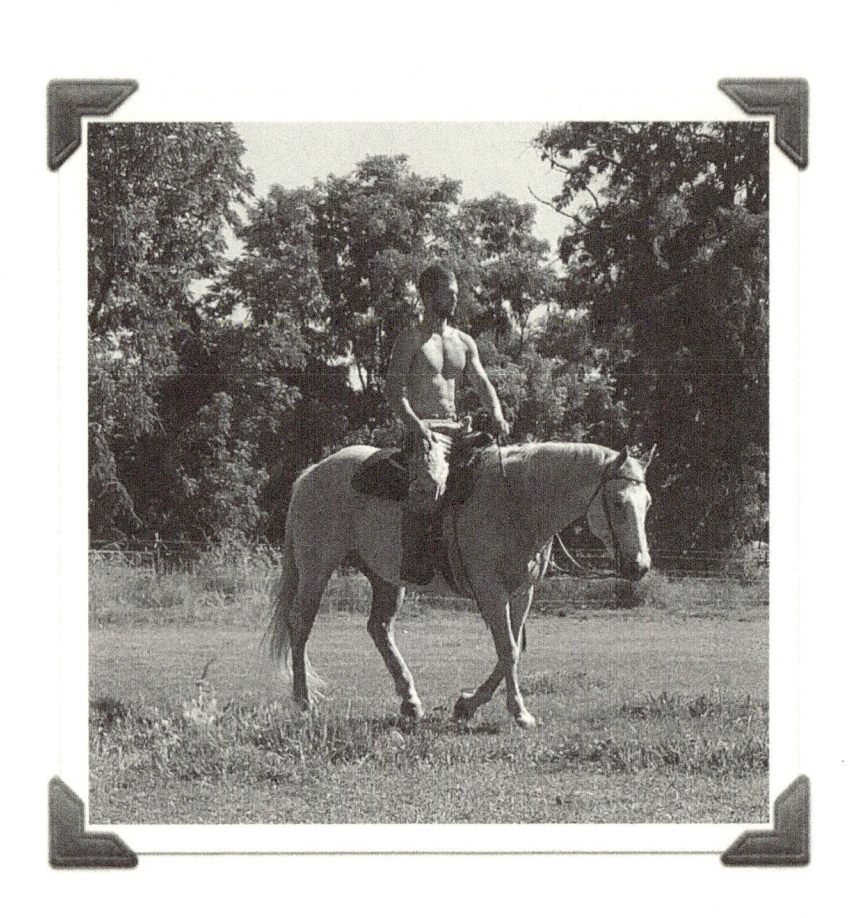

I soak up sunshine whenever I get a chance, especially in the winter when it's harder to get enough vitamin D.

SUNSHINE, FRESH AIR, EXERCISE, GOOD FOOD, GOOD BOOKS, ENOUGH SLEEP, AND FRIENDSHIP.

My family laughs, 'cause I'll be stripping down as I go *outside* to exercise, and putting more clothes on when I come back *in*.

ENJOY THE ADVENTURE CALLED LIFE

Also take cod liver oil (Carlsons lemon flavored is pretty good, no fishy taste), and get grass-fed butter if you can.

LACK OF VITAMIN D CAN CONTRIBUTE TO FATIGUE, ACHINESS, LOW IMMUNE RESPONSE, PHYSICAL WEAKNESS, WEAK BONES, ANXIETY, AND DEPRESSION.

SUNLIGHT IS ONE OF THE EASIEST AND CHEAPEST MEDICATIONS. JUST DON'T BURN!

Massage

I like a form of Russian massage that I learned through Systema. Primarily we use the arch of the foot to press on our partner's body while they lay on the floor. You can also press big muscles, or knots, with your toes, heel, or the ball of your foot.

Using the feet to massage allows deep pressure, but spread over a larger area than work with hands, and you can scale it from lightly resting one foot on your partner to full on standing on them.

Do <u>not</u> stand on joints!

Check out Vlad's video "The Combative Body" available from Systema HQ at RUSSIANMARTIALART.COM
Also look for a Systema Instructor qualified to teach you.

My family also likes Ortho-bionomy, developed by Dr. Arthur Pauls, D.O. and taught by Terri Lee.

It is a system of gently accentuating tensions, so your body will recognize and then relax and release them.

Society of Ortho-bionomy: ORTHO-BIONOMY.ORG

Terri Lee: SOLDANCIN.COM

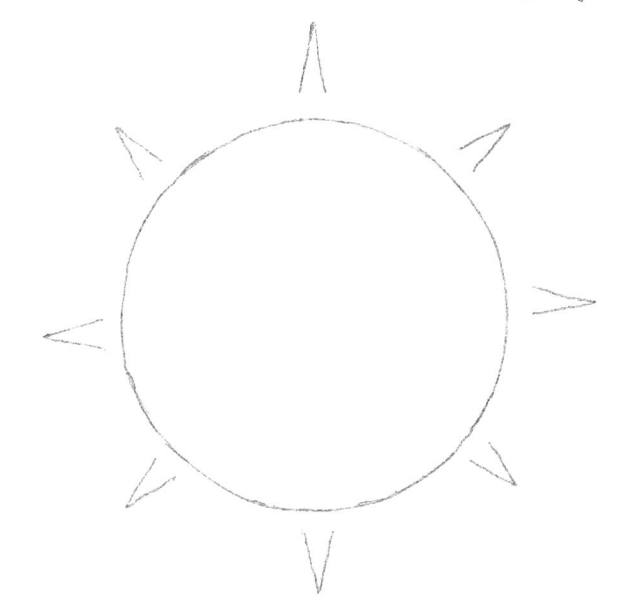

ACV

Raw apple cider vinegar is amazing stuff. It aids digestion, boosts energy, balances pH, lowers blood sugar levels, kills harmful bacteria, and can help with weight loss.

WE EVEN FEED ACV TO OUR COWS - FOR HEALTH & ATTITUDE

I routinely add raw ACV to my drinking water. I like to have a quart size glass jar on a shady part of our kitchen counter, and every time I fill it up I add a couple teaspoons of raw ACV. To me, it tastes better than plain water. That quantity isn't enough to make it sour, it just adds a pleasant tang.

You can also use lemon or lime juice if those are more appealing. Or run all three in a cycle.

A pinch of salt can be helpful in the heat of summer on days I'm out working and sweating a lot.

Water

I like drinking cool room temperature water; it feels like less of a shock to my system than chilled, or especially iced, water. And I like letting it sit in glass or ceramic; I've heard that the water molecules form or charge in a healthier way than when in metal.

I do run a metal waterbottle for traveling and adventures. Doesn't have the same flavor or feel as glass, but it's durable and far better tasting than water in plastic, especially that single use plastic crap. Don't fall for the 'ease' of single use plastic; our landfills are overflowing and our oceans are drowning by our laziness. Also cheap plastic leaches unhealthy chemicals into your water (and food).

I MADE A PARACORD WRAP FOR TEXTURE & EASIER CARRY. 35 FT OF CORD!

Get a decent steel or glass waterbottle; keep track of it, and reuse it!

I've had the same glass quart jar since I was 14, and the same metal waterbottle since I was 18.

GET UNLINED STAINLESS STEEL.

Fasting

Fasting provides a myriad of benefits: mental clarity, spiritual awareness, endurance and fortitude.

> HOW CAN WE TRULY FEAST, IF WE NEVER FAST?

Fasting allows your body to rest from constantly digesting the latest load of food you shovelled in, and provides slight discomfort for you to test yourself against.

How do you function without your normal food? Grumpy? Tired? Reach deep and work on yourself.

Healthy cells have plenty of reserves to survive several days without food. Sick and mutated cells are the ones that scream for food and water first, but if you push through the initial hunger, they will die off and leave you stronger.

Be a little careful, I did a heavy workout at the end of a 24 hr fast and kind of crashed my blood sugar; my energy dropped and I came in and ate and ate. Counter-productive

But have confidence that you are far more resiliant than you realize. Christ said, "Keep a cheerful face. do not let others know you are fasting."

I like 24 hr fasts, though you can go far longer.
I eat a light meal at 6pm, skip breakfast and lunch, and eat lightly again at 6pm the next day.
My goal is to do this once a week.
Just set a specific day as a fasting day in your weekly schedule.

Foraging

Wild food is rich and nutritious. Many plants we think of as weeds are actually time honored sources of food and medicine for those with the eyes to see and knowledge to appreciate the gifts they give.

What is a "weed"? just a plant growing where a human doesn't want it. Many have deep tap roots which pull up a wide spectrum of minerals and nutrients, and a vibrant energy for life. Those pass to you when you eat those plants. You can pick them fresh out of your yard, and they're incredibly filling.

STOP THINKING "WEEDS" AND YOUR LAWN BECOMES A SALAD BAR.

"Eat dandelions for power and plantain for health. Eat them both as much as you can."

— Jamie Lippiatt

I'm still learning and have a long way to go in integrating large quantities in my regular diet.

For now, there are several plants I graze on when I see them on my daily field walks.

Dandelion: a few leaves contain more calcium than a glass of milk. Dandelions provided strength and energy to Resistance fighters on Crete, on the run from the Nazis after they had kidnapped the Nazi commanding officer.
In the spring you can harvest them anywhere, but in the heat of summer they're much more tender when grown in the shade. It also helps to harvest after they've been watered or rained on. Otherwise they can be kind of tough and bitter.
I leave a patch unmowed in my yard, and put a sprinkler on them for a couple hours the night before I want to harvest.

Plantain: long leaf or round leaf. Plantain is a drawing agent, good for stings and infections. You can apply it topically - just chew up a couple leaves and put the pulp on the sting or wound.
Or when you eat it, it draws out toxins internally and cleanses your organs. I used it in conjunction with yarrow on scrapes and mat burns that got infected; one was pretty bad, my whole knee was hot and swollen, but the plantain/yarrow cleared it right up.

Yarrow: antibacterial, antimicrobial, good for stings, and one of the fastest natural ways to stop bleeding.
Beautiful plant. I always keep an eye out for it, whether I'm on the farm, high in the mountains, or exploring a foreign city. It grows everywhere, just look.

I saw one of my instructors cut himself on a flint blade, pretty deep. But his wife ran out, picked yarrow from just outside the lecture hall, chewed it up on her way in, and applied it to the cut. Bleeding stopped moments later.

Purslane: one of the few plants that have a full complement of Omega-3 fats; usually you find those in animal products — grass-fed eggs and dairy, grass-finished beef, ocean-run salmon.

If you pick it in the heat of the day or around noon, it has a very refreshing tang with a hint of citrus. Excellent snack or addition to a salad.

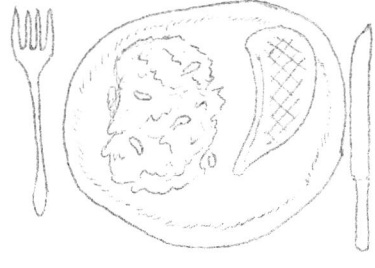

Wild rosehips: packed with an accessible form of vitamin C, and ripening in early winter as other sources wither. The cold doesn't bother these at all.

I pick a couple every time I walk by, all through the winter and spring. They have a bunch of seeds inside with some rather stiff hairs, so nibble carefully, but the fruit is sweet and tastes somewhat like dried cherries.

Mother Nature is a beautiful system that has been designed to provide lavishly for her children.

FURTHER RESOURCES:
TOM BROWN'S FIELD GUIDE TO WILD EDIBLE AND MEDICINAL PLANTS — TOM BROWN, JR

THE WILD WISDOM OF WEEDS — KATRINA BLAIR

THE DANDELION HUNTER — REBECCA LERNER

The Wild Thirteen
or the 13 heroes
From 'The Wild Wisdom of Weeds' by Katrina Blair

Well worth a read!

- Amaranth
- Chickweed
- Clover
- Dandelion
- Dock
- Grass
- Knotweed
- Lambsquarter
- Mallow
- Mustard
- Plantain
- Purslane
- Thistle

These grow around the world, wherever people live.

They thrive in disturbed soils, and are easy to identify.

I like to mix wild greens into a salad with lettuce or spinach, it mellows the stronger flavors of wild food, but you're still eating it and benefitting. —A.

Maffetone Method

I first heard of the Maffetone Method in Natural Born Heroes and I really like it.

It involves a 2 week "reset" where you don't eat any sugars or processed carbohydrates, or even sweet fruit or starchy vegetables.

This teaches your body to burn fat as fuel and provides long sustained energy, instead of depending on sugar rushes with their inherent crashes.

After the reset, you can add sugars and carbs back into your diet, but maintain the awareness of how they make you feel.

Even a couple years after doing the reset, I still feel the benefits.

I have some carbs and sugars, but often skip a meal here or there and don't even miss it.

BASIC FOOD GUIDELINES
LOOK UP philmaffetone.com
FOR MORE SPECIFICS

YES

- raw & cooked vegetables
- tree nuts (except peanuts & cashews)
- fruit & berries
- beef, turkey, lamb (grass finished & organic)
- fish (wild caught)
- eggs
- cream } organic
- unprocessed hard & soft cheese } &
- yoghurt & kefir } grass-fed
- oils (olive, avocado, coconut > corn, safflower, canola)

NO — at least use moderation and discipline

- All sugar
- sweets & desserts
- all non-calorie sweeteners — natural or artificial
- bread
- pasta
- corn
- energy bars
- processed meats & cheeses
- fruit juice
- all soda & diet drinks
- sports drinks

THE 2 WEEK RESET IS SOMEWHAT DIFFERENT AND MORE STRICT.

Diet, or No-diet

I don't believe there is one optimal super-diet for all people everywhere.

Pay attention to your body. Cut out junk food and as much sugar and processed carbohydrates as you can, and then see what appeals and feels right as you eat it.

I know people who have used both vegan regimes and carnivore diets as a cleanse or reset with great success.

However, I'm skeptical of either for long-term; I think it is difficult to get the full spectrum of nutrients we need, in the proper quantities.

And I know a couple guys who had pretty severe health problems after a poorly planned vegan diet.

Do your research.

Optimally, diet follows a cycle with the seasons.

I eat more fresh fruit, greens, and light food in the warm months when hydration and electrolytes are primary concerns, and more root vegetables and stews and broth in the cold when dense supplies of stored energy are important for generating heat.

I always eat a lot of healthy fats and animal protein (grass-fed dairy and eggs, grass-finished beef), but it's worth noting that somewhere around half the energy in fats and protein is converted to heat as you digest it. In the summer it's best to eat those foods in the evening as the day cools.

One of the best things you can do for your health is to learn to cook for yourself as you gain awareness and appreciation for quality ingredients; how they taste, how they were grown, and then how how the food makes you feel.

Organic

Organic standards are a set of requirements that prohibit the use of petro-chemical pesticides, herbicides, and fertilizers, and artificial growth hormones and antibiotics.

It's important to know your source, and know your farmer.

There are factory farms that are certified Organic, but it's still factory farming and the quality of life for animals and the quality of products are both in question.

This doesn't mean don't buy Organic. It's still an important step, far better than conventional practices, and voting with your dollars sends a message.

Just remember, the message gets louder, and the quality of food better, the closer to home you can buy.

Search out both local AND Organic

With a small scale local Organic farm there is much more transparency.

My family owns and operates a 160 acre farm where we raise grass-finished Organic beef.

We host farm tours periodically, and welcome people contacting and visiting us. We'll walk you out to the pasture, point out the wide diversity of plants our cows graze (up to 40 different grasses and broadleafs with different nutritional, mineral, and medicinal strengths), and introduce you to our animals. They all have names.

We care for animals with dignity and respect, and steward the soil for the health of the planet, the animals, and ourselves.

Grass fed & grass finished

Animals are healthiest when they are outside in the sunshine and on green grass.

Cows are designed to eat grass and forage, not shovel in pounds of grain. A grain diet creates an acidic environment in their stomach that allows harmful bacteria and E. Coli to propagate. When cows eat grass, as intended, the acidic environment simply doesn't exist.

Cows eating grass produce high Omega-3 fats; the same healthy fat found in ocean-run salmon.

Make sure to look for grass _finished_ beef; some operations pasture their cows most or some of their life, and put them in a feedlot for the last sixty or ninety days, reversing the health benefits of grass feeding.

THE SAME PRINCIPLE APPLIES TO DAIRY, IT'S HEALTHIER FROM ANIMALS IN THE SUN AND GREEN.

CHICKENS AND OTHER POULTRY DO NEED SOME GRAIN. BUT YOU CAN ALWAYS TELL THE PASTURE RAISED EGGS BY THEIR BRILLIANT YELLOW YOLKS.

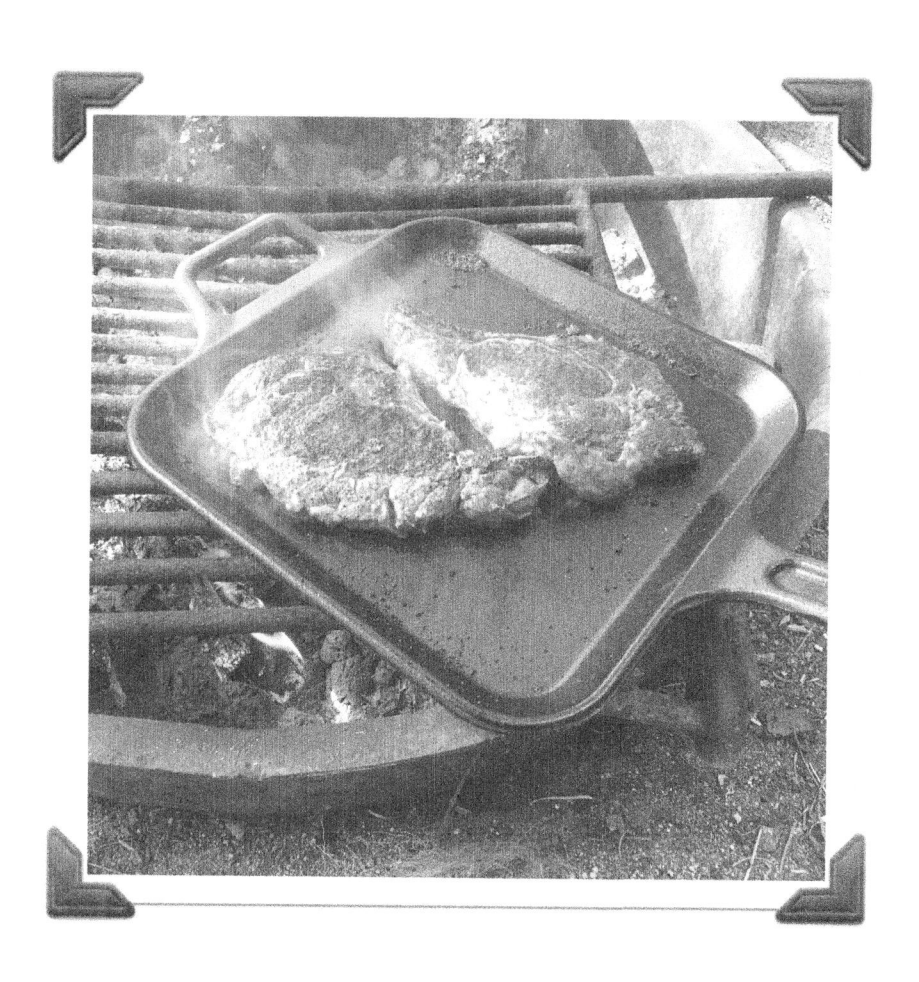

Healthy Fat!

Your brain is comprised of a large percentage of fat.

Healthy fats are essential for brain function, joint health, sustained energy, and overall wellbeing.

FASTING & ACV ARE HELPFUL TOOLS FOR DETOX.

We actually isolate and store toxins in fat cells to protect our vital organs. This is why exercise, while important, sometimes isn't enough. We have to clean up our diet and allow the body to detox. Many people find they lose excess weight when they switch to a diet high in healthy fat.

Saturated and unsaturated fats are good for you provided they come from a clean Organic source. Avoid transfat 100%!

GET ALL ORGANIC ⟹

Good sources include grass-finished meats, pasture raised eggs, grass-fed raw dairy, many kinds of nuts and seeds, avocadoes, and olive oil, coconut oil, sunflower seed oil, flax seed oil, avocado oil, and cod liver oil.

Fats are slower to digest but provide deeper satisfaction and satiation, and long-lasting sustained energy.
Sugars and carbs hit your bloodstream too fast and leave you with a sugar rush, and then a crash and a craving for more.

America isn't fat because we eat a lot of fat (the fat-free fads have seen to that), but because we are highly sugared and grain-fed like cows in a feed-lot, and have no sense of portion control.

Do you want to eat like a grain-fed cow bellying up to the feedbunk, ready for slaughter?

Or like a jaguar, lithe and lean; on the hunt, with danger in the eye?

Pat Mac – Diet Advice

Eat when you're hungry, stop _before_ you are full. Eat to about 70% – what if you had to go _right now_ to save yourself or someone else?

Don't be a human garbage can! Eat real food! Anything in a bag or a box is a product.

Shop around the periphery of the grocery store. If you venture into the center, go with a purpose – salt, pepper, coffee, olive oil. Don't get sucked into the cereal aisle.

In addition, consider that water is the number-one dietary supplement. Powerslam a quart every morning to start the day.

"ROCK 'N' ROLL!"

PATRICK McNAMARA IS THE AUTHOR OF 'SENTINEL' AND COMBAT STRENGTH TRAINING! HE RUNS SOME NEAT RANGE DAYS, AND HIS INSTAGRAM IS SOLID. FOLLOW @tmacsinc

"You cannot divorce strength from health."
— George 'The Russian Lion' Hackenschmidt

"For me, health goals are exciting. It's about growth, not trying to change yourself because you don't like who you are.
Treat your body like a garden — a constant work of love.
Be the gardener of your own body and cultivate radiant health."
— Stephen Deitrich, Forest Warrior Arts

"Do the best you can until you know better. Then when you know better, do better."
— Maya Angelou

Part 3:
Further training and thoughts

"Overcoming yourself is the hardest victory because the enemy is just as strong."
— Vladimir Vasiliev

"Relentless learning is the hallmark of a great teacher. Those who think they know it all are already obsolete. If you choose to teach others, it is your duty to keep learning."
— Dan Edwards

"We are what we repeatedly do. Excellence then, is not an act, but a habit."
— Aristotle

"God sends the wind, but man must raise the sails."
— St. Augustine

"A harmless man is not a good man. A good man is a very dangerous man who has that under voluntary control."
— Jordan Peterson

"If you want peace, prepare for war."
— Vegetius

"Speak softly and carry a big stick."
— Theodore Roosevelt

"It is better to remain silent and be thought a fool, than to speak and remove all doubt."
— Abraham Lincoln

Obi-wan Kenobi:
A devastating warrior who'd rather not fight. A negotiator without peer, who frankly prefers to sit alone in a quiet cave and meditate.
— Matthew Stover, 'Revenge of the Sith' novel

EDC — Every Day Carry

Pockets:
- Knife — Benchmade Griptilian
- Light — Streamlight Microstream
- Paracord — 12 ft

Jump Pack:
- Water Bottle
- First Aid Kit
- Trauma Kit — Tourniquets, Pressure Dressings, Chest Seals
- Tracker Knife
- Multi-Tool
- Water Filter — Sawyer Mini
- Sunflower Seeds and Almonds
- Fire Kit — Bic Lighters, Flint & Steel
- Paracord — 100 ft
- Foil Emergency Blanket
- Light Windbreaker
- Poncho
- Wool Hat
- Shemagh
- Fingerless Wool Gloves

Never walk away from home ahead of your axe and sword. You can't feel a battle in your bones or foresee a fight.
— The Hávamál

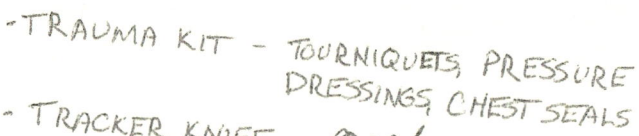

When I put together these kits, I kept a list in my wallet and just tried to pick up an item or two every couple weeks.

Be Prepared.
— Boy Scout Motto

VEHICLE KIT

CONSOLE:
- LIGHT - J'S TACTICAL
- TRAUMA KIT - TOURNIQUETS, PRESSURE DRESSINGS, CHEST SEALS

There is no bad weather, only bad clothing.
— Swedish Proverb

These lists have grown over several years as I see what I use and what I lack, and get new ideas from other people

ASHTRAY:
- BANDAIDS
- BATTERIES - AAA & AA
- BIC LIGHTER

GLOVE BOX:
- BATTERIES
- SPARE HEADLIGHT BULB
- PRESSURE GAUGES (2x)

DOOR POCKETS:
- ICE SCRAPERS (2x)
- MAPS

TRUNK BOX:
- BOOSTER CABLES
- TOW STRAP
- ROAD FLARES (4x)
- TIE DOWNS
- PARACORD - 100 FT
- 2 QTS OIL
- 1 GAL WATER
- BIC LIGHTERS (4x)
- WOOL BLANKET
- TOWEL
- 8x10 TARP
- PAPER TOWELS
- TP
- SPETSNAZ SHOVEL
- DUCT TAPE
- GARBAGE BAGS

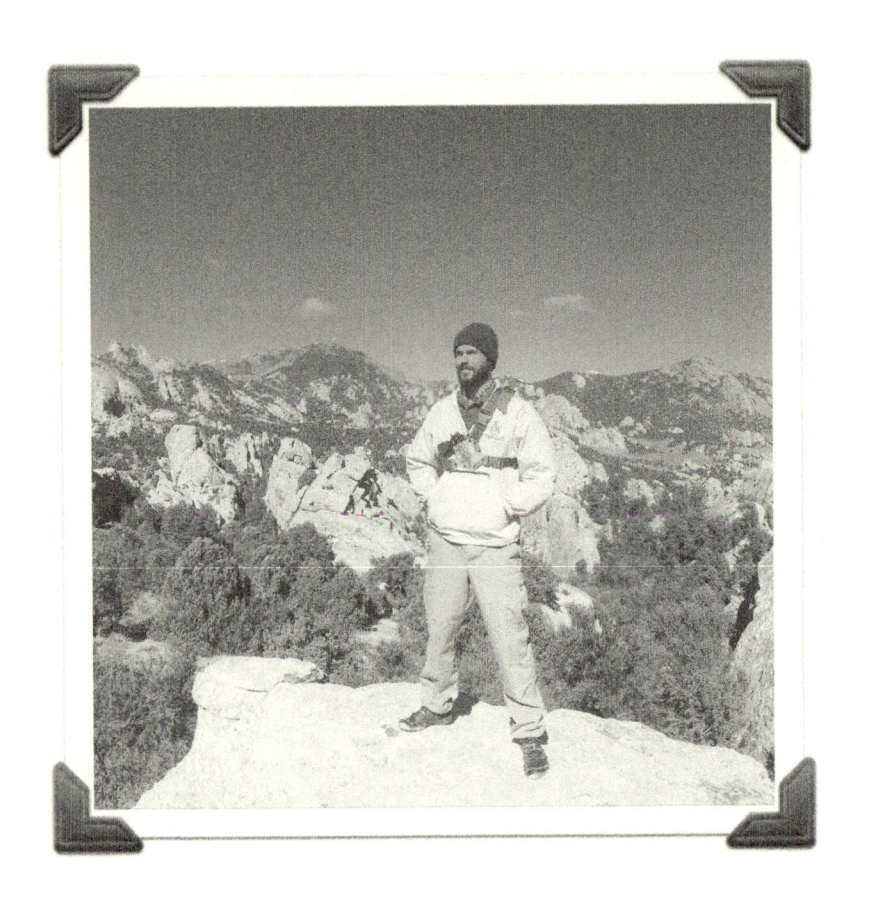

Being prepared means being ready to withstand and survive disaster, but also to fully enjoy unexpected opportunities.

In mid-October 2018, my brother put together a trip to City of Rocks with some friends, and I decided to join them. It had been a warm October, and he had been there in August when it was quite warm, so I didn't think about the park being at 6800 ft. I just grabbed my normal camping and EDC gear and we headed out.

This could have been a very chilly trip, however it turned out to be an excellent gear check and a really fun time! We run 0° sleeping bags, thermarest pads, and good tents; so usually sleep warm and well.

Then in the morning, in the frost and cold breeze at sunrise, I pulled out the windbreaker, wool hat, and gloves I carry, and layered with my standard wool shirt was tolerably warm and content.

We spent a gorgeous weekend hiking, scrambling and climbing in some fantastic country.

Learned two things:
1. remember to check weather forecasts.
2. my gear set up is working well. Onward!

100 Skills
Every Man Should Know
ArtofManliness.com

1. tie a necktie
2. build a campfire
3. hang a picture
4. shine your shoes
5. treat a snakebite
6. read a book
7. survive a bear attack
8. wet shave
9. parallel park
10. paddle a canoe
11. negotiate/haggle
12. fix a leaky faucet
13. treat a burn
14. tell a joke
15. predict the weather
16. do a deadlift properly
17. recite a poem from memory
18. grill with charcoal
19. perform CPR
20. throw a spiral
21. sew a button
22. split firewood
23. find potable water
24. change a flat tire
25. break down a door
26. take the perfect photo
27. sharpen a knife
28. change a diaper
29. give a speech
30. navigate with a map and compass
31. unclog a toilet
32. buy a suit
33. swim the front stroke
34. shake hands
35. treat frostbite
36. iron your clothes
37. practice situational awareness
38. do a proper pull-up
39. build a shelter
40. grow your own food
41. cook eggs
42. make small talk
43. identify poisonous and edible plants
44. do a front dive
45. shuffle cards
46. hunt
47. properly pour beer
48. perform the fireman's carry

49. open a bottle without an opener
50. cast a fishing line
51. speak a foreign language
52. drive in snow
53. perform the heimlich maneuver
54. ask a woman on a date
55. always know north
56. fell a tree
57. hitch/back up a trailer
58. play poker
59. write in cursive
60. throw a knockout punch
61. make pancakes from scratch
62. skipper a boat
63. dress for the occasion
64. shoot a bow and arrow
65. drive stick shift
66. do a proper push-up
67. pick a lock
68. mix two classic cocktails
69. field dress game
70. play one song on the guitar
71. use a chainsaw properly
72. do a squat properly
73. cook steak
74. entertain yourself (without a smartphone)
75. change your cars oil
76. whistle with your fingers
77. shovel snow
78. carve a turkey
79. tie a bowline
80. ride a horse
81. give a good massage
82. get a car unstuck
83. break a rack of pool balls
84. make a logical argument
85. cook bacon
86. write a letter
87. shoot a gun
88. make a toast
89. jump start a car
90. know how to dance
91. brew the perfect cup of coffee
92. tie a tourniquet
93. know two cool uncle tricks
94. fillet a fish
95. calm a crying baby
96. ride a motorcycle
97. hammer a nail correctly
98. cook a signature dish
99. make a fire without matches
100. tell a story

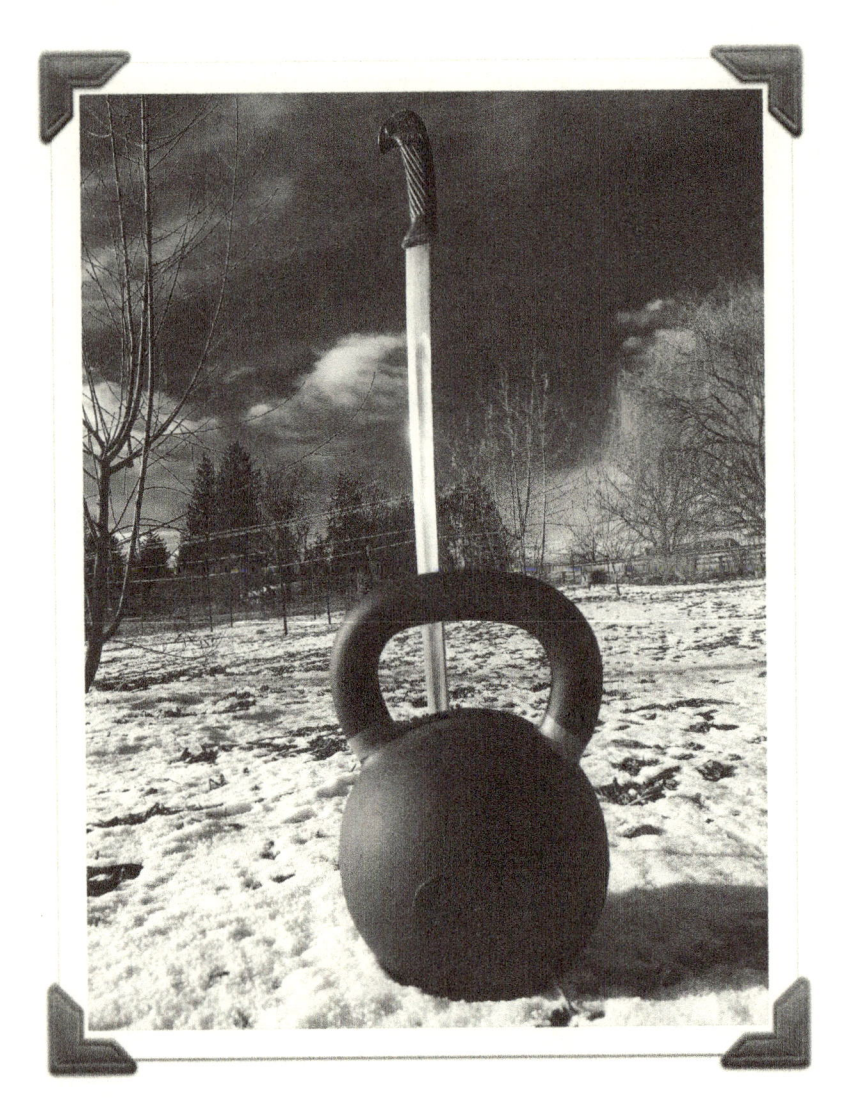

Why do we do what we do?
For the strength to carry the weary,
the skill to defend the weak,
the will to act,
the ability to make a difference.

"You may think that you are completely insignificant in this world.
But someone drinks coffee from the favorite cup that you gave them. Someone heard a song on the radio that reminded them of you. Someone read the book that you recommended, and plunged headfirst into it. Someone smiled after a hard day's work, because they remembered the joke that you told them today. Someone loves themself a little bit more, because you gave them a compliment.
Never think that you have no influence whatsoever. Your trace, which you leave behind with every good deed, cannot be erased."
— Unknown

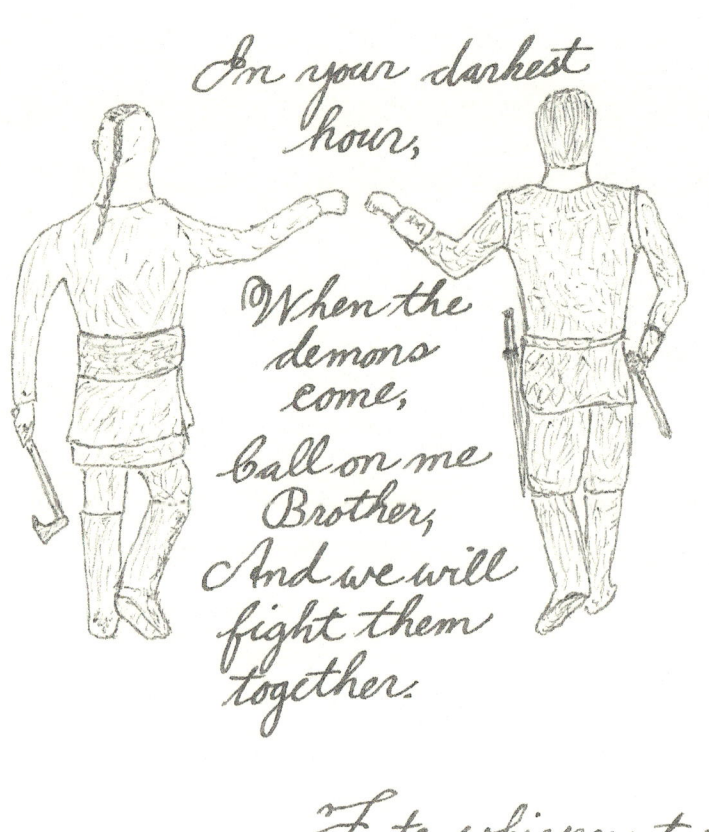

In your darkest
hour,
When the
demons
come,
Call on me
Brother,
And we will
fight them
together.

Fate whispers to the warrior
"You cannot withstand the storm."
The warrior smiles
and whispers back
"I am the storm."

If by my life or my death
I can save you,
I will.
— Aragorn

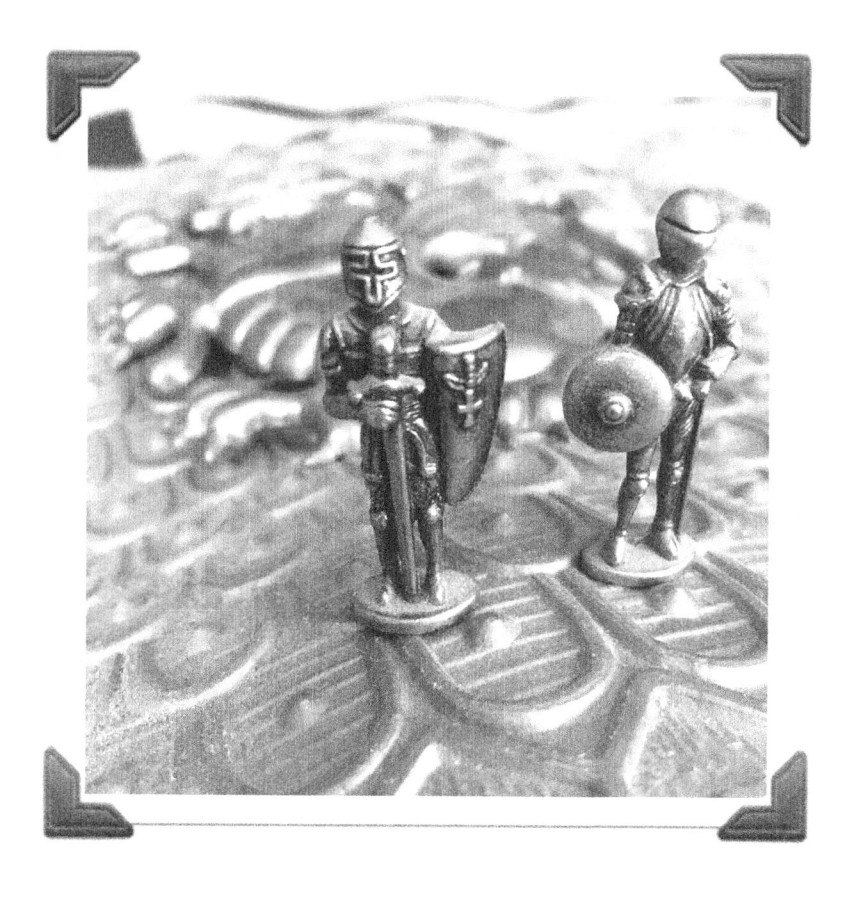

Forgive me my failings,
the brother I did not reach
in his hour of need.
Teach me to see, to know, to act.
Teach me to be the protector,
the pathfinder, the guardian,
the Scout.

"Every child should learn to swim, ride, and fight."
— Helio Gracie

"The society that separates its scholars from its warriors will have its thinking done by cowards and its fighting done by fools."
— Thucydides

"How do you want to lose? By a big throw, or a series of penalties? This is the essence of banzai, 'I will win, or I will die; but I will <u>not</u> sit by on the sidelines.'"
— Rex

"Always assume that your opponent is going to be bigger, stronger, and faster than you, so you learn to rely on technique, timing, and leverage, rather than brute strength."
— Helio Gracie

"If you win, do not boast of your victory;
and if you lose, do not be discouraged.
When it is safe, do not be careless;
and when it is dangerous, do not fear.
Simply continue down the path ahead."
— Jigaro Kano

"Be quick to listen
and slow to talk,
quick to move
and slow to anger."
— Vladimir Vasiliev

"If you think, you are late.
If you are late, you use strength.
If you use strength, you tire.
And if you tire, you die."
— Saulo Ribeiro

"Are you a martial artist?
Strive to make the art
your own.
Be an artist."
— Matt Hill

"The pen isn't mightier than the sword. Pens don't win battles. And swords don't write poetry. Mighty is the hand that knows when to pick up the pen and when to pick up the sword."
— Anonymous

"Accept that there are things in this world we can never explain and life will be understandable. That is the irony of life. It is also the beauty of it."
— The Gift of Rain

"He who knows the art
of the warrior is not
confused in his movements.
He acts and is not confined.
Therefore Sun-Tzu said,
'He who knows himself
and knows his enemy
wins without danger.
He who knows the heavens
and the earth wins out over all'."
                  -Eiji Yoshikawa
                      'Musashi'

"Gracefulness is not an
unmasculine trait.
As a quality, it combines
playfulness, relaxation,
and power.
It is the perfect balance
of caution, joy, and assertiveness.
The fool laughs at grace.
The warrior embodies it."
                  -Stephen Deitrich
                  Forest Warrior Arts

"Awareness begins inside and expands outward.
Hypervigilance is an external skill.
Careful not to confuse the two.
One leads to self awareness, humility, and an expanded vision of life; the other can blind us to our self deceit and shrink life down to a series of threats."

— Gene Smithson

Awareness

"Situational awareness" gets a fair bit of air time in tactical and semi-tactical training courses, but there is so much more to life than always "scanning for threats" or "watching your back."

We should learn to see, really see, and hear, and taste, and smell, and feel, and sense, and know.

Live, really live.

Enjoy the good things. Walk with your head up and your shoulders back and drink it in.
Seek out challenges and enjoy the adventure.

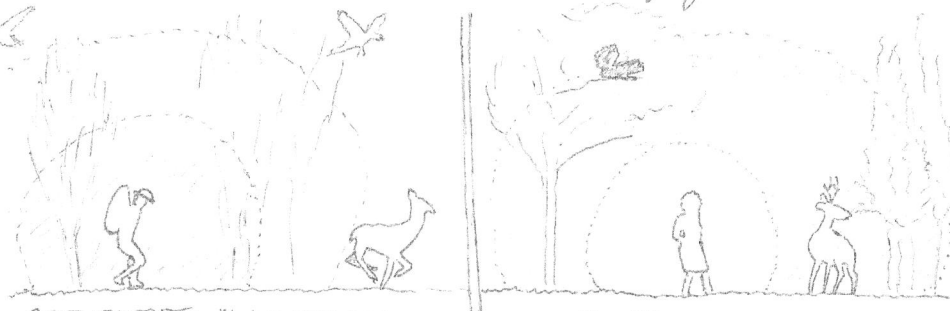

ART EXCERPT: "WHAT THE ROBIN KNOWS" BY JON YOUNG

At Tracker School, the Sacred Question of the Apache Scouts is "What happened here? What is this teaching me?"
You may not know the answer, but simply asking a question helps you observe more deeply.

Did you see the Red-tail hawks circling above that field? Did you smell the rain coming on the wind and how it lifts the scent of sagebrush with it down from the hills? Why is that car going slow? Did you hear the Mourning Doves on the first day they're back in the spring, and notice how they're consistently 3-4 weeks behind the Eurasian Collared Doves? What is that cat hunting in my backyard? Why is that person limping, if injury, where, if carrying something, what? Which way is north?

What route do the squirrels always take to get from tree to tree? Is it going to rain soon, how does the air feel, and what do the birds and animals say? Is that person armed and/or capable, or not? Did you see the deer grazing on the hillside above the road or the osprey sitting in the tree down by the river? What color was the noisy truck that sped by? How quietly can I move on this surface or in this environment? How long until sunset?

ASK!

Learn your area's baseline, or normal activity, and then the anomalies and oddities will stand out.

"Give yourself a test. Pause for a moment and answer these simple questions: What kind of cloud was in the sky the last time you were out? Which way was the wind blowing? How many different kinds of wildflowers can be seen from your front door? How many different birds have you heard today? Where is the nearest rabbit, owl, deer, coyote, or fox?

If your awareness is as sharp as it could be, you'll have no trouble answering these questions."

— Tom Brown, Jr.

I HAVE A LOT OF WORK TO DO! —AFD

Sit spot

Find an area you like where you can sit quietly and watch the flow of life around you. This can be a space deep in a wild area, or in a park, or in a coffee shop, or your own front steps.

Tom Brown says you need to sit at least 30 minutes so the disturbance of your entry will die away and baseline activity resume.
Konstantin Komarov said even 7 minutes will help you improve drastically.

I like to make a cup of hot tea and go sit on a glider chair on my deck. I can hear the ebb and flow of bird calls and cars going by and occasionally a cow talking in the field. Sometimes a cat will come sit with me. I want to quietly enjoy my tea, and then when it's gone it's time to move on to the next thing.

Survival Awareness

Tracker School notes

Always see the beauty, first & foremost. Then the utilitarian aspects of the landscape: bowdrill wood, cordage material, hunting & trapping areas, water sources, etc.

Keep your mind alive.

Tips for Observation:

Be relaxed. Look around, use your neck.
Relax physically and mentally.
Use all your senses.
If something seems out of place, check it out. Carefully, of course.
Spot the animal before it spots you.
Pay attention to air movement/wind; drop some dust to see.
Cover anything that shines: watch, glasses, face.

Don't focus on one thing, scan the
    landscape.
Stay out of the rut, it's so easy to get caught
Look through the closest trees, through
the brush, and beyond.
Look for parts of the animal.
Check heights and placement of animal
head / body for trap size.
Horizontal lines are odd. Check.
Transition areas - meadow to woods,
    field to untilled area, streambank, etc.

Awareness
Live your life toward.
Sacred Question: "What happened here?"
             "What is this teaching me?"
Ask the why about everything.
Solve the mysteries, but first you
    have to see them.
Being with humans creates "time"
being alone in solitude is it's own
rhythm, into eternity.

Fox walk

Place the outside of the ball of your foot down first. Roll your step in so your whole foot is on the ground, then shift your weight.

① → ②
③ full weight

Keep your weight back so you can reach forward with each step instead of falling onto it.

You can speed this up to a run, a swift gentle fox run is refreshing. Or if you need to be extra quiet, slow down and drop into a crouch, make one step per 66 seconds, and you may omit putting the heel down.

Try to move in a level manner, not bobbing your head up and down with each step.

EARTH-TIME: 4 COUNT PER STEP

YOU CAN SEE MORE WHEN YOU SLOW DOWN. ENJOY THE JOURNEY.

Moving this way utilizes your tendons and ligaments to absorb the impact of each step the way we were built to.
But if you are used to heel-stomping in thick cushioned shoes, this method of walking will take some practice and getting used to.
And it won't work very well with many modern shoes.
Go barefoot whenever you can, and look up Xero shoes or some kind of minimalist trail runner.

If you do have to wear thicker soles, roll from the outside of your heel diagonally up to your big toe. Called the Stone Stalk, this is also the quietest way to walk across rocks, sand, and gravel.

Stone Stalk

RATHER THAN PROTECTING YOUR JOINTS, THICK SOLED SHOES ARE ACTUALLY AN UNSTABLE PLATFORM THAT PUTS UNDUE STRESS ON YOUR TENDONS AND CONTRIBUTES TO TORN ACHILLES AND OTHER SPORTS INJURIES.

Several years ago I took the Scout class at Tracker School, and it includes a lot of stealth work and night exercises.

They taught us, beyond the fox-walk and stalking steps, how to roll across short spaces so as to look like a raccoon from a distance, or how to mimic a deer's movement by bending forward and staggering the cadence of your steps.

And it was beautiful to watch the instructors cross sand roads at a run; throwing handfuls of sand from bags they carried, right into each footprint as their foot left, obliterating their tracks

Late one night, my team had completed our objective and was headed back to camp. We had just turned off of a road, onto a path to cut through the swamp, when we heard a vehicle.

Most of our eight man team was ahead, just a friend and I were still close to the road covering our tracks.

We did a quick "sink and fade" into the underbrush, but the vehicle pulled up right beside us and some volunteers got out.

Thinking we were made, we jumped up and bounded down the path, bent over and staggering our steps. No one shouted or shot any bottle rockets after us.

The next morning we told one of the instructors the story and he smiled and said the volunteers had just stopped to empty a cooler, and then came into their camp talking about how they'd scared up a bunch of deer right by the road. We smiled.

At the end of that Scout class as we were packing up, I was heading down the main path on an errand, and met one of the Shadow Scouts going the opposite way.
We smiled, and he said "Take care of yourself."
I said "I will." And kept going.
A few minutes later I was headed back the other way and met him approaching again. Again we smiled and he said "Take care of yourself."
This time I said "I will, so I can take care of others."
He paused, and his grin got wider, and he said "You got what you needed."

    I never saw him again that I know of, but that exchange has stuck in my memory.

The Sacred Question:
"What happened here?" and "What is this telling me?"

Scout training lasts a lifetime.

Always be in the Scout Mindset, how would you get on top of that building? where could you hide in that parking lot? how would you move silently through that brush? or leave no tracks? The Game is always on!

WARRIOR — HEALER
△
SCOUT

Look, listen, learn = live

Always seek intensity over mediocrity.

Safety, Security, and Comfort are euphemisms for Death.
Think of a time you more than remember, but relive.
Bet you weren't safe, secure, or comfortable; but you were damn well alive.

Train hard
walk soft

The Fox and the Skunk

I went running barefoot early one May morning to make a quick irrigation change.
I saw a small fox hunting rockchucks, and then almost tripped on a skunk as he meandered into my path.
He dove one way, I dove the other and everyone was fine.
Perhaps I run too quietly and ought to carry bells, but I don't think so.

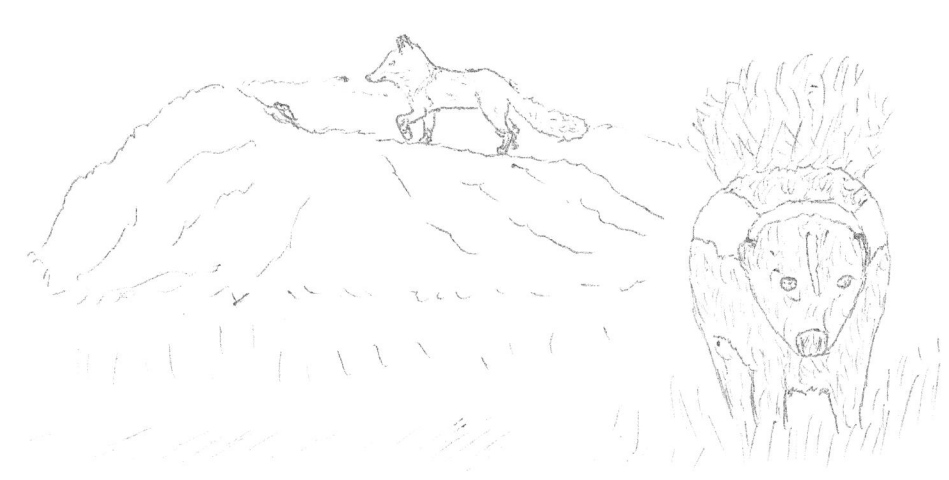

"Waiting to start training in martial arts until you're in "better shape" is like a child not going to school until they are "smart enough."
— BJJ world

"Violence is rarely the answer, but when it is, it's the <u>only</u> answer."
— Tim Larkin
'When Violence is the Answer'

Stout heart is better than strongest sword. Yet, the bold oft are beaten who have blunt weapons.
— Völsungasaga

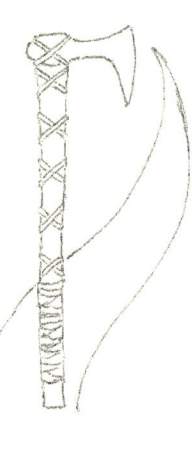

"I tend to focus on martial.
I like it. I'm good at it.
So here is an argument for art.
Violence and crime rates continue
to fall, while crude, purposeful
ignorance and meanness rise.
More and more people packed
into smaller and smaller spaces
and rudeness and vulgarity
seem to rule.
So. Maybe the art part....
the moving beautifully, the slowing
down.... the attention to courtesy
and calm are valuable pieces
of the pie. Still.... best to
keep the sword sharp."
— Gene Smithson

It is better to be a warrior
in a garden, than a
gardener in a war.
— Chinese Proverb

Tannaz Sepehri

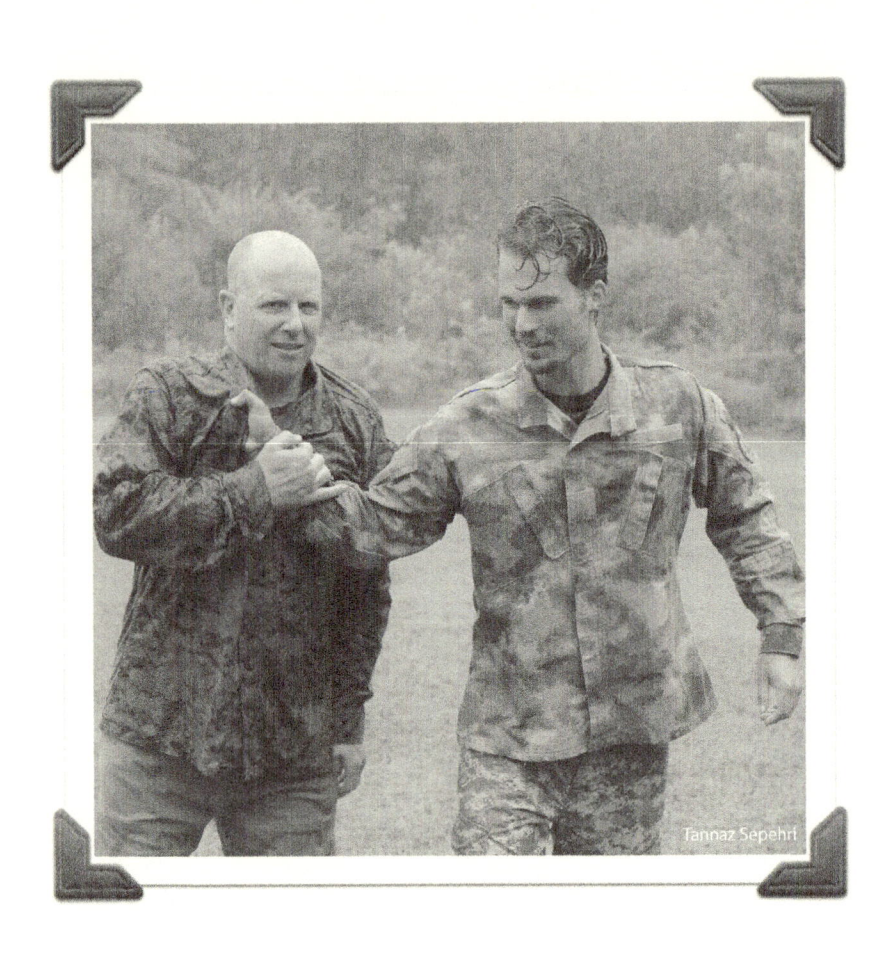

Systema

Systema is beautiful as a fighting system, an art, and a way of life. I've struggled to write about it; one has to feel it.

Systema has been described both as one of the most brutally effective fighting systems, and one of the most humane martial arts. The aim is to destroy the attacker's aggression and desire to attack, not destroy the attacker.

There are three major areas of training: combative skill, physical strength and health, and spiritual mastery. Together, they build overall well-being for body, mind, and spirit.

COMBAT SKILL
TAKING HITS
SPARRING
FLUIDITY IN MOTION

OVERALL WELL-BEING

BREATHWORK
CALISTHENICS
COLD WATER DOUSING
CLEAN DIET

SPIRITUAL MASTERY
HUMILITY
MENTAL FORTITUDE

Taking strikes, slow calisthenics, and dousing in cold water allow humility and self mastery to grow and pride to be chipped away.

As your spirit grows stronger you do not feel as sorry for yourself, irritations diminish, and you discover longer endurance and more freedom in movement. Giving and receiving strikes brings you face to face with reality. You confront fear and release tension. How terrible is it to be hit? Sometimes it is bad. And sometimes we worry needlessly about something that is well within our capacity.

And it's hard to be self-centered and proud during a set of 15 push-ups on a single breath-hold. Everything in you becomes focused on survival. Pride creates tension, tension burns oxygen, and that dimishes your survivability.

When an unstoppable force meets an immovable object, people get hurt.
Don't be an immovable object, or you will break.
Did he hit you?
So what? MOVE!!
You may then find an opportunity to share a strike with him.

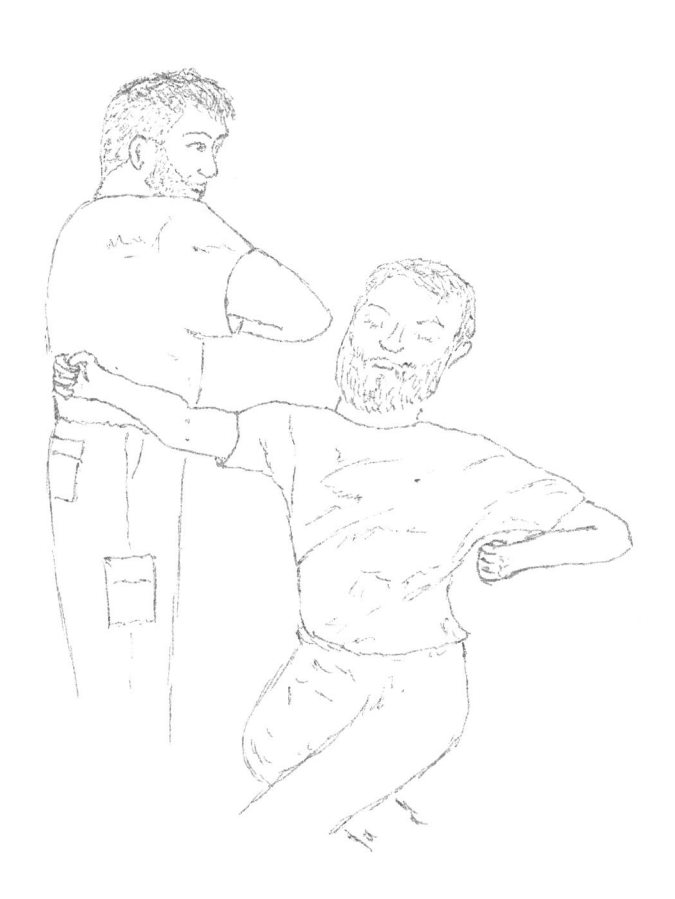

"DON'T BE A TOUGH GUY."
       -VLAD

When you learn to relax and release excess tension and fear, you move into a state of alert freedom. You are able to shrug off heavy strikes, or let the impact go right through your body without damage.

Whether receiving strikes or dealing them, let the power flow through you. Do not get caught up in the tensions in your body or the fear in your psyche.

Practice this with slow work, both partners working at ¼ or ½ speed, sparring, but using fists and feet to push rather than strike or kick. Accept your partner's fist on your body or face. Allow the gentle force of his push. And explore how it moves your body, how you react, how he reacts and whether you are now positioned for a counterattack. Check your distance, and send the power he just gave you right back into him with a push of your own.

Look for points of tension or muscles that are supporting the body and/or the movement.
Those are your targets. Push there. A simple push will have effect, and when you move to strikes, a seemingly gentle strike will have nearly explosive results.

Approach training and combat as just another job to do. Don't emotionalize it. Be calm, be cool, and just do your work. Mikhail Ryabko, the head of Systema world-wide from Moscow, says, "butter your toast."

TRUST THE TRAINING

Calmly deal with the situation as it comes. You don't pull out a cavalry saber and hack your toast to pieces, just butter it. Keep the same mentality when dealing with an aggressor.

Systema has no ranks or belts,
or forms or rules.
Everyone trains together, in a largely
freeform environment.
Each person has a unique approach
or response and you can learn
from and with one another.
A teacher is a guide, someone
further down this path.

My teacher, Vladimir Vasiliev, is an amazing man. Exhibiting nearly effortless mastery in motion, he always has a grin and a kind word, and heavy fists.

He spent ten years in one of Russia's elite units of Spetsnaz. His unit learned the Ancient Russian Martial Art - Systema. They recognized its combat efficiency and spiritual strength which helped them deal with the stresses of Afghanistan and Chechnya and largely reduce their cases of PTSD.

Because of Vlad's relaxed response to attacks in demonstrations or seminars some people think it's fake or staged. Those that actually train with Vladimir usually change their mind. Look up the video titled "HIT DIFFERENT" (on the Systema Vasiliev youtube channel) of someone launching a high kick at his head, and his response. The kick ruffles his hair, but not his presence.

If you can, visit Systema HQ in Toronto. People come from all over the world to train for a few days, weeks, or months. You will be warmly welcomed.

Systema HQ also has several books in print and a large library of instructional videos available on DVD or to download at RUSSIANMARTIALART.com, as well as a directory of schools and instructors around the world.

The motto of Systema is "Poznai Sebia" which is translated as Know Thyself. Know yourself: your capabilities, your innermost thoughts, your shortcomings, your strengths. And know for yourself. You have to feel and explore and find it for yourself and make it your own.

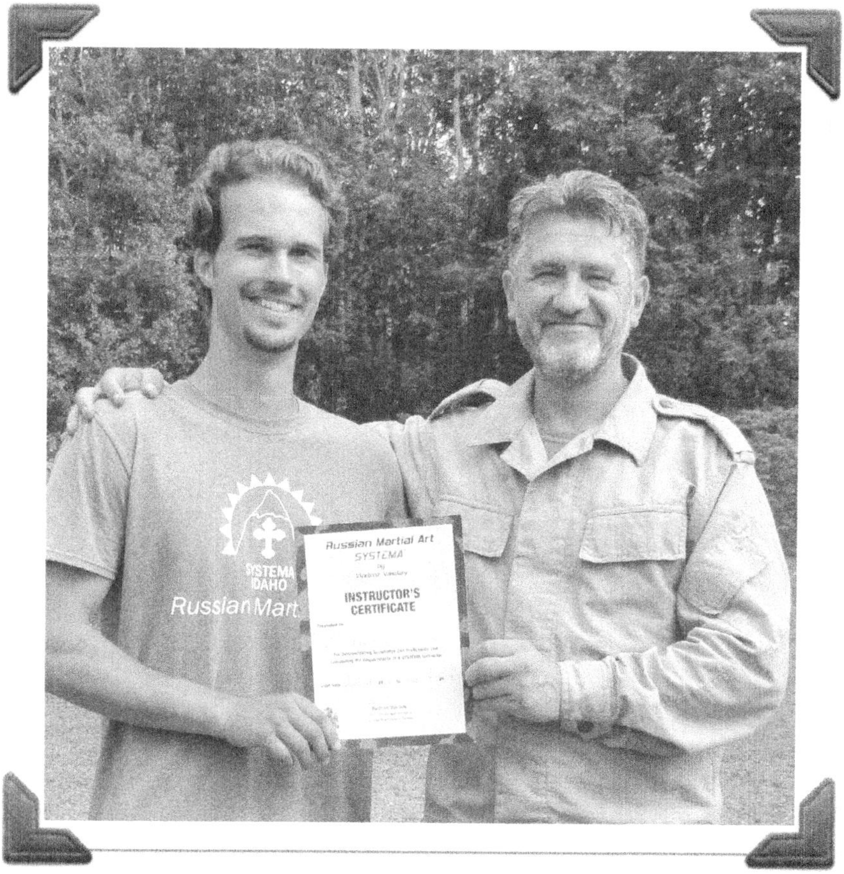
SYSTEMA
IDAHO
Russian Mart
Russian Martial Art
SYSTEMA
INSTRUCTOR'S
CERTIFICATE

Judo Notes

Your goal should be to put your opponent on the ground; it doesn't much matter how they get there, 'techniques' are specific ideas for accomplishing that goal.

Learn and apply them correctly, they are distilled application of momentum and leverage.

But remember the goal:

1. Put him on the ground
2. Take dominant body position
3. Do your judo, no fear

PRACTICE PERFECTION DURING UCHI-KOMIS. ACCEPT 'GOOD ENOUGH' IN MATCHES AND RANDORI.

"Judo helps us to understand that worry is a waste of energy."
— Jigaro Kano

"If you are tense, you are fighting two people, yourself and your opponent."
— Vladimir Vasiliev

- MAXIMUM EFFICIENCY, MINIMAL EFFORT - workout every day, train every day. Prepare yourself so in competition - or life when a task arises - you can simply call on strength and skill, rather than straining and stressing.

- MUTUAL BENEFIT AND WELFARE - take care of your training partners so we can practice again and again and again. If you practice a technique 100 times and your partner practices it 100 times, you'll both be 100 times better than someone who dumps his partner once and breaks him.

- HIGHEST PERSONAL DEVELOPEMENT - push yourself. Train with the biggest and most skilled people you can find; the people who can exploit your flaws, and in doing so, help you correct them.

Golden Rules of Grappling

1: Be the guy on top.
2: When on top, stay on top.
3: When on bottom, have a guard you shall not pass.
4: Never forget Rule 1. Easily forgotten due to the seductive and rewarding nature of guard.

— Prof. Chris Haueter

Learn to Flow Roll — @jiu_jitsu_brotherhood

Most people have only one speed when rolling — flat-out.
The best grapplers are able to shift gears according to the situation that is presented. They can roll light when their opponent rolls light and amp it up if he pushes the pace. By removing the competitive element from sparring, flow rolling helps you learn how to use these "gears".
It's also a fantastic drill for improving cardiovascular endurance, timing and agility.

"Work on kuzushi (breaking balance).
Pull them off _balance_,
don't pull _them_.
Then relax so they can't read you.
Strength should be elastic,
like a rubber band.

Close the distance. It feels uncomfortable to be closer to your opponent, but your work is ineffective from too far away. Get close, stay loose!

"It's a pretty dance,
but in this dance,
you _have_ to lead."
     -Rex

"The skillful judoka does not oppose your action directly, but he just introduces sufficient "grit" in your works to make your action sluggish and only just fall short of your aim; otherwise he must be at least as powerful and as fast as yourself." -Moshe Feldenkrais, HIGHER JUDO

Trust the training. Trust the technique. It's an interesting mix of putting the effort in, but also just setting it up correctly and then mentally stepping back and letting the work flow.

5 parts of a throw:
- kuzushi - break balance
- tsukurai - fitting, or position
- kake - enter throw
- nage - throw
- hime - support

MUSHIN — NO MIND.

"THERE IS NO TRY. ONLY DO, OR DO NOT."
— YODA

AND ALSO TRY, AND THINK, AND TRY AGAIN, AND WORK, UNTIL YOU SUCCEED.

☼ 8 directions of off-balance. have a throw for each direction.

During randori (free practice):
Against a weaker player do not let up, but practice and perfect a wider range of techniques. Against an equal, bear down, attacking and applying your most successful techniques. Against a stronger opponent, concentrate on defense, but also look for opportunity to apply the pressure of an aggressive attack. In every case, seek to make each movement a work of art.
— Judo Textbook

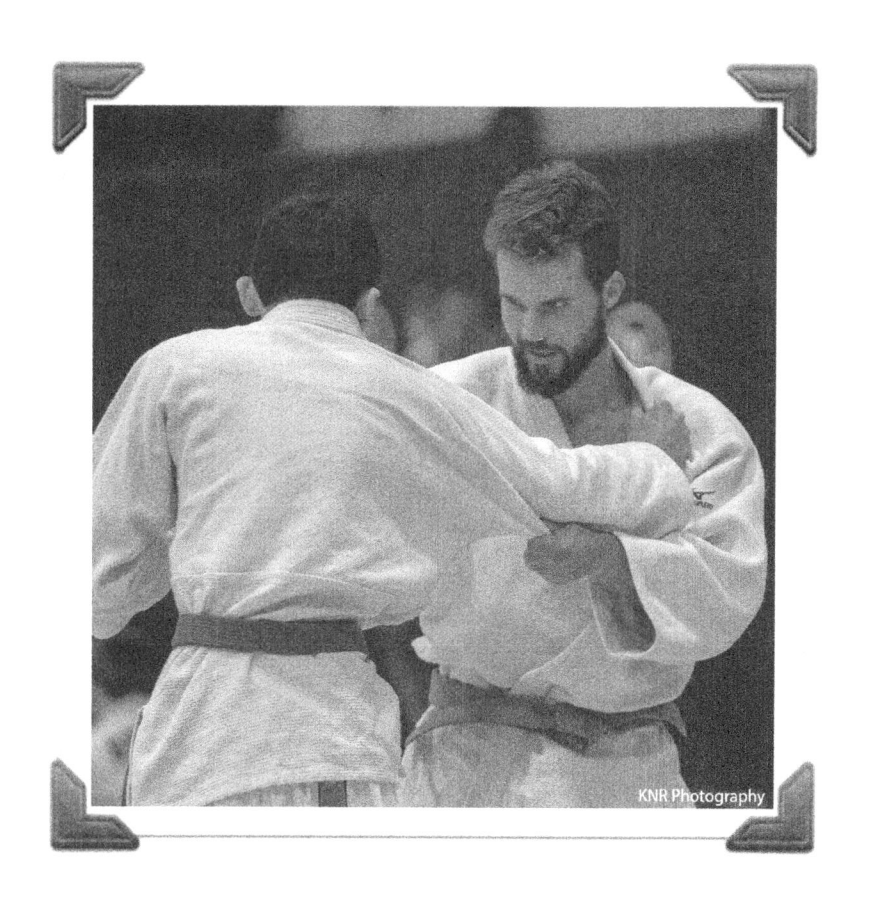

Develop the ability to act first
and think and talk about it later.
— Judo Textbook

Overwhelming strength
can only be used against you
if you try to oppose it.
— Judo Unleashed

Judo Notes: Tank vs. Sniper

I'm a light guy; I'm 6' tall but my fighting weight is about 155 lbs. My buddy Jacob is about 5'11" and 230 lbs.

One of our Senseis came by as we were practicing and said, "Jacob, you are like a tank. Heavily armored, and big weapons, but limited fuel supply. Aaron, you are like a sniper. Light, fast, precise, and lots of endurance. How does a tank win? By continually pounding the sniper's position and/or then running him over. But focus on attack and finish the match before your fuel runs out and you gas yourself out. How does a sniper win? By keeping moving until the tank is out of gas, then picking off the crew. Keep attacking to keep him off balance, but don't go strength to strength."

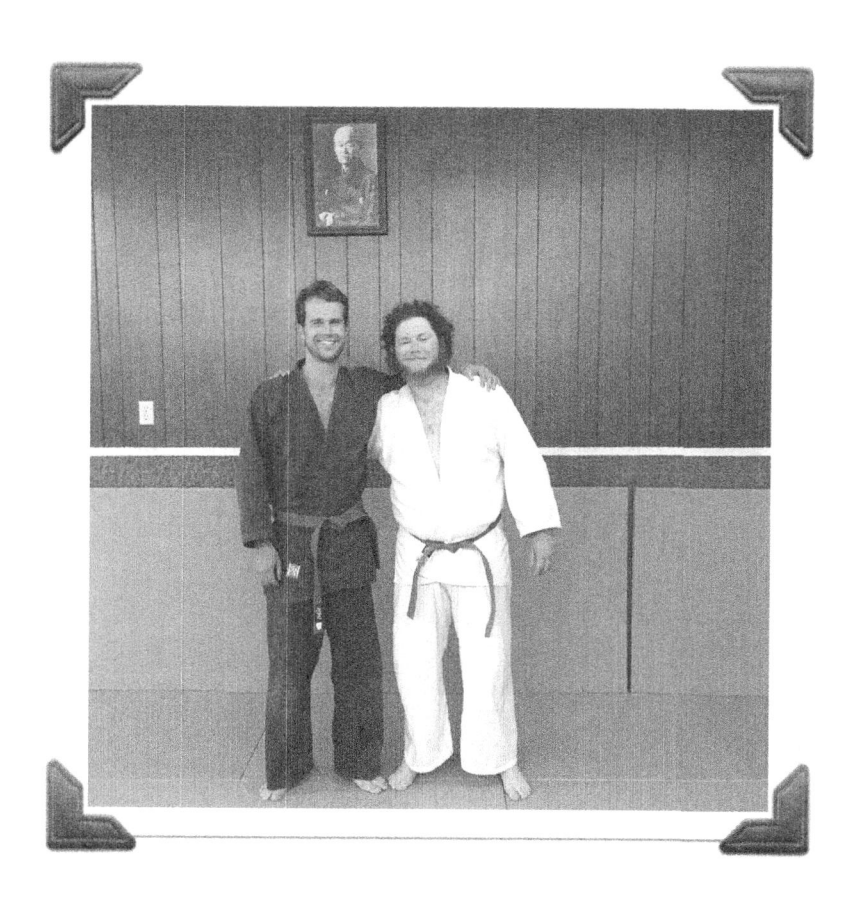

Fixed Mindset vs. Growth Mindset

Fixed Mindset:
- Avoids challenges
- Ignores feedback & critique
- Intelligence & talent are fixed
- Less effort
- Gives up easily
- I am a failure
- Feels threatened by success of others
- I will never improve

Growth Mindset:
- Embraces challenges
- Learns from feedback & critique
- Intelligence & talent can be developed
- More effort
- Keeps trying & never gives up
- Persists in the face of setbacks
- Inspired by the success of others
- I will learn

The Growth Mindset
@jailhouse_strong

The growth mindset dictates that no one is born a winner or a loser, but rather a chooser. This means you can be the winner if you want to be; you don't have to come into existence a certain way.

In other words, it's not a matter of smart vs. dumb, but learner vs. non-learner.

This mindset views challenges as tools to help someone grow rather than a bad omen.

The growth mindset finds feedback constructive and recognizes that effort is necessary. In short, growth mindset is a "yet" mindset. For every cause there is an effect, choices are a matter of free will; you are the master of your fate.

Developing a Growth Mindset
@failhasestrong

1. Embrace belief
Believe in yourself and your capabilities and you will open up your potential to achieve your goals.

2. Embrace challenges
Use challenges as a means to get better.

3. Embrace hard work
Rather than something to be intimidated by, hard work is a necessary ingredient in pushing yourself to your full potential.

4. Learn from criticism
Receiving criticism isn't easy, but it is important. Find the value in it and use it to better yourself, no matter how harsh.

5. Be inspired by success
Rather than stewing in envy of others' success, use it as inspiration for your own. Instead of looking at the negatives of a situation, look for the opportunity for your own success.

6. Have a white belt mentality
Recognize that you can learn from anyone, anywhere, at any time.

7. Cultivate a sense of purpose
Start with the "why." The "how" will come later.

8. Believe in heroes
Seeking inspiration in those you look up to. Use this to motivate yourself to reach their level and beyond.

9. Develop self-awareness
Be able to reflect honestly on your progress. Know that you only have as much potential as you allow yourself to have. Are you at 85 percent growth / 15 percent fixed mindset or vice versa? Either way, you can begin shifting your current mindset to one of total growth right this very second. What will you accomplish once you do?

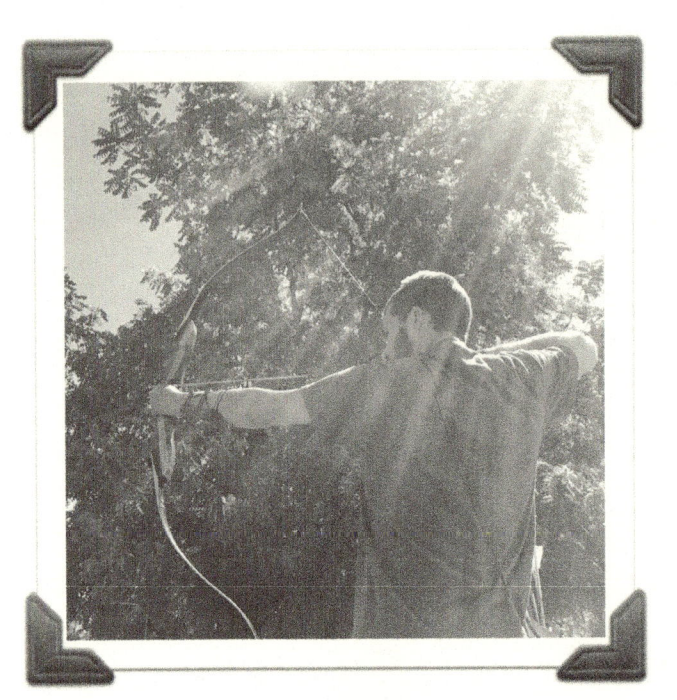

Drenched in sunshine and bowsong.

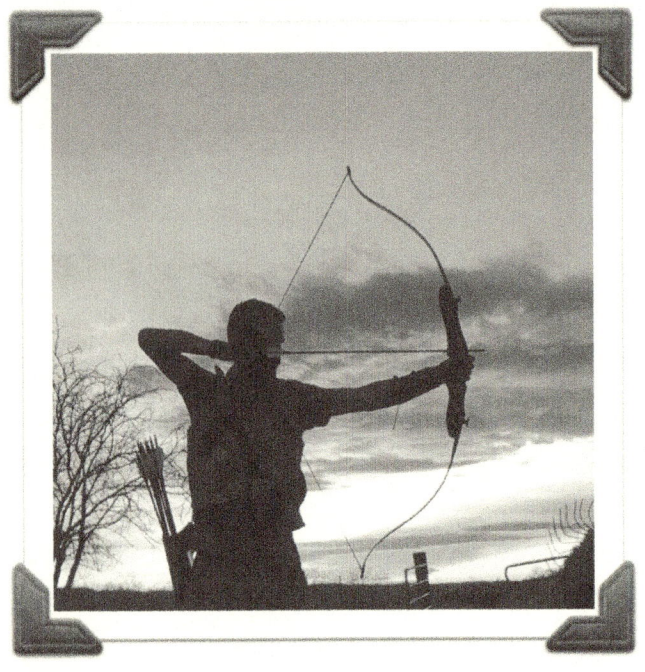

Evening stillness, and the song of the bow, and the staccato of each arrow striking home.

Archery

I'm not a great archer, I don't practice often enough, or consistently. But I love it.

There is something calming and peaceful in the draw and release, the great song of the bow, and the arrow whirring downrange to impale the target.

"NOTHING CLEARS A TROUBLED MIND LIKE SHOOTING A BOW."
 — FRED BEAR

HE'S RIGHT.

When I asked Emmanuel Manolakakis the Systema Archer, for recommendations for a beginner, he suggested getting a 25 or 30 lb recurve; sufficient power to be worthwhile but light enough to allow hours of sustained practice.

And that's what I did.

Buying new, a 30 lb recurve and a dozen arrows plus accoutrements set me back around $300 US.

Three years later after many, many volleys sent downrange, it is definitely worth it!

The Celt, by Charles Fox

Bronze, to tip the wild rose fronds,
the arrows of the Celt.
Owl feathered, somewhat weathered
from cold rains he has felt.

A bow of yew, shaved and true,
blessed by Druid song.
A tattooed shaft with leather haft,
oiled and buffed and strong.

'Neath full moon, when lovers swoon,
this man of ages gone
Blend and meld, his magic held
in his weapons and his brawn.

With hefty axe he follows tracks
but the bow he keeps in hand,
For dangers howl and often prowl
this ancient wooded land.

Put bow and arrow in his barrow
when his time is done,
Remember him, this ancestral whim,
the Celt, the mystic one.

"SO LONG AS THE NEW MOON RETURNS IN HEAVEN BENT, SO LONG WILL THE FASCINATION OF ARCHERY KEEP HOLD IN THE HEARTS OF MEN." —MAURICE THOMPSON

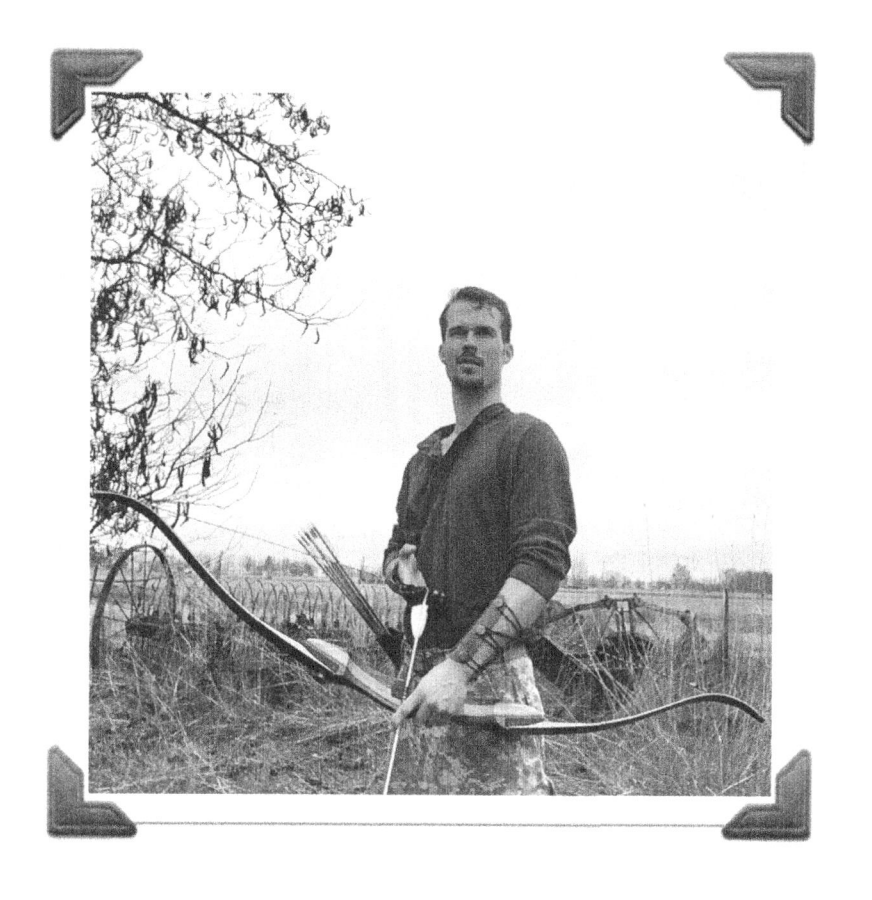

Silver grey rain, bow song, peace.

"In archery, we have something like the way of the superior man. When the arrow misses the center of the target, he turns around and seeks for the cause of his failure in himself."
 -Confucius

Gunfighters Prayer

Lord, make me fast and accurate.
Let my aim be true and my hand
faster than those who seek to destroy me.
Grant me victory over my foes
and those who wish to harm me and mine.
Let not my last thought be,
"If only I had my gun";
and Lord, if today is truly the day
You call me home...
Let me die in a pile of empty
brass.

"Just because you have a gun does not mean that you are armed. The mind is the final weapon. All else is supplemental."
- Pat McNamara

"Fast is fine, but accuracy is final. You must learn to be slow in a hurry."
— Wyatt Earp

"If you are in a profession that is not tactical in nature, when you come to the range you should consider working from concealed. Maybe doing mag changes from your pockets, etc., and not throwing on a couple thousand dollars' worth of fancy gear."
— Pat McNamara

"Be religious about doing a little PT every day, treat dry-fire as your daily devotional to the gods of war, and get to the range once or twice a month to verify your dry-fire practice."
— John Mosby
'Clandestine Carry Pistol'

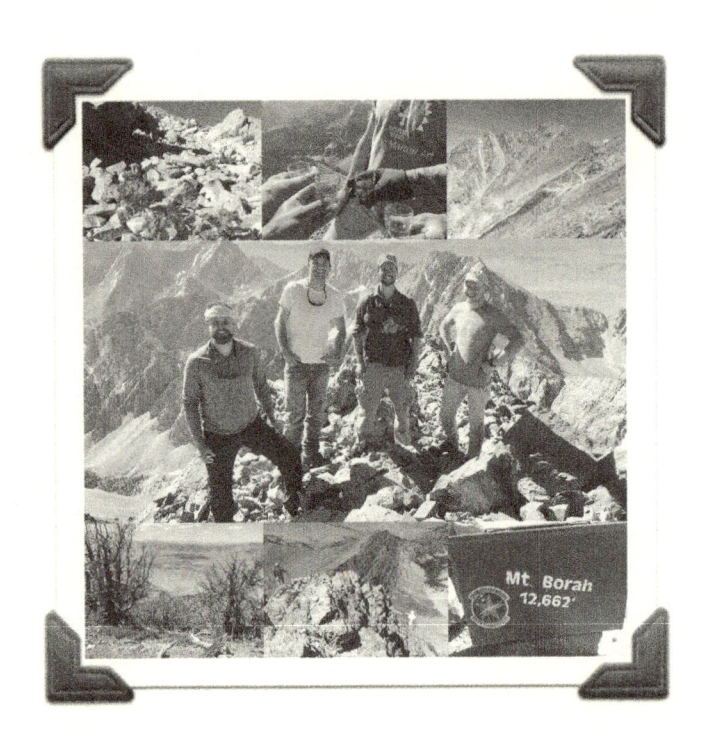

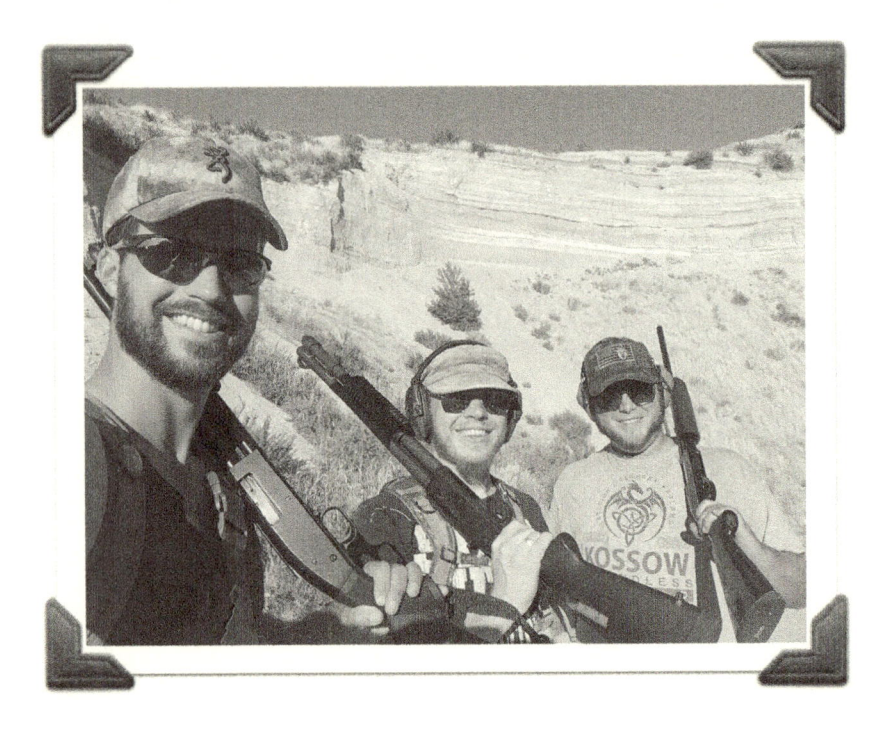

Tribe

We live in an era of digital connection, and personal isolation and increasing desperation.

It is imperative to have people in our tribe, our clan, our war band, people we can gather with regularly.

We are built for community.

These are people we reach to for help, and the ones who join with us to celebrate and rejoice.

While social media and the internet are useful tools, and I draw a lot of inspiration and joy from interactions with my brothers and teachers across the globe, there comes a time to put down the damn phone, turn off the computer, and walk out into the sunshine and free air and find the red-blooded friends who also are stirring from the digital apathy and finding their way into the light of day.

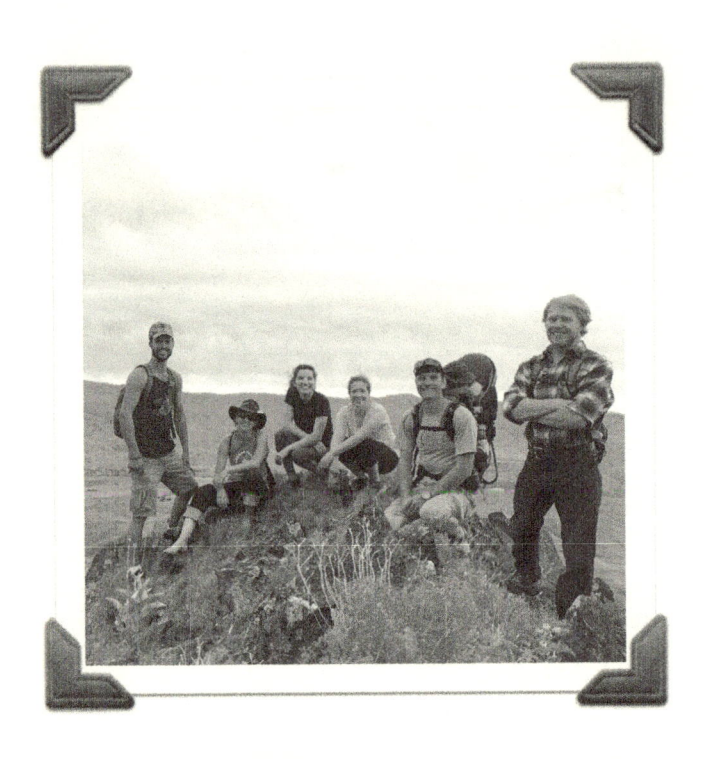

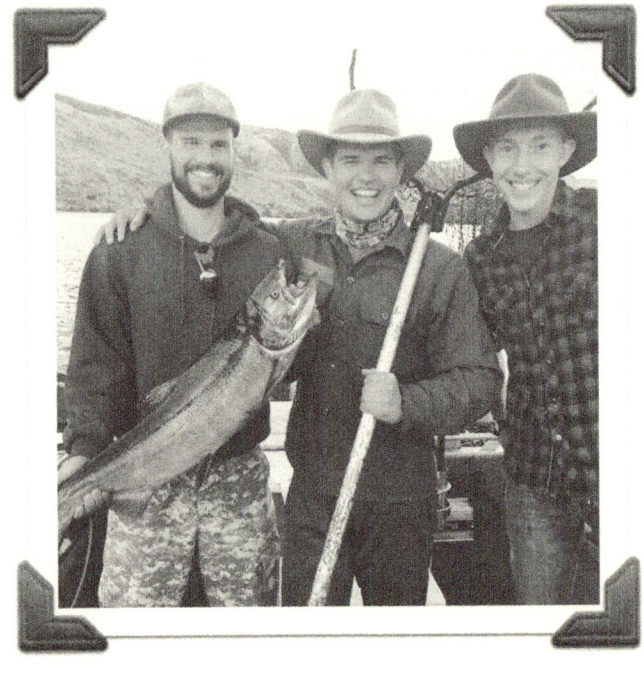

Eating together, breaking bread together, can be a powerful step in building relationships, especially when you can assemble early and cook together. Talk over your perceptions of current events, history, good books or movies you found thought provoking, revel in the glories of your last adventure, or start planning the next one.

Dinner and watching good movies are great, but move soon to adding some more active pursuits; see how you work together, forge your team. Go for a hike, build something together, go shooting, workout, or do some specific training like going to a climbing gym or taking up a martial art.

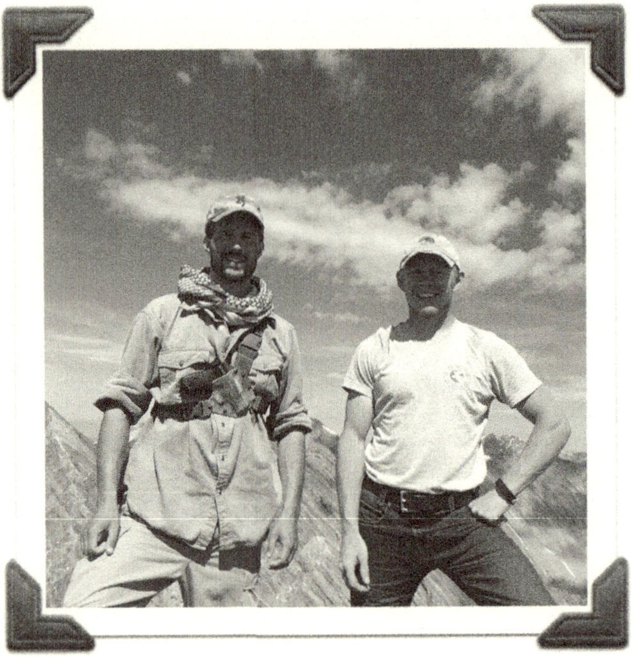

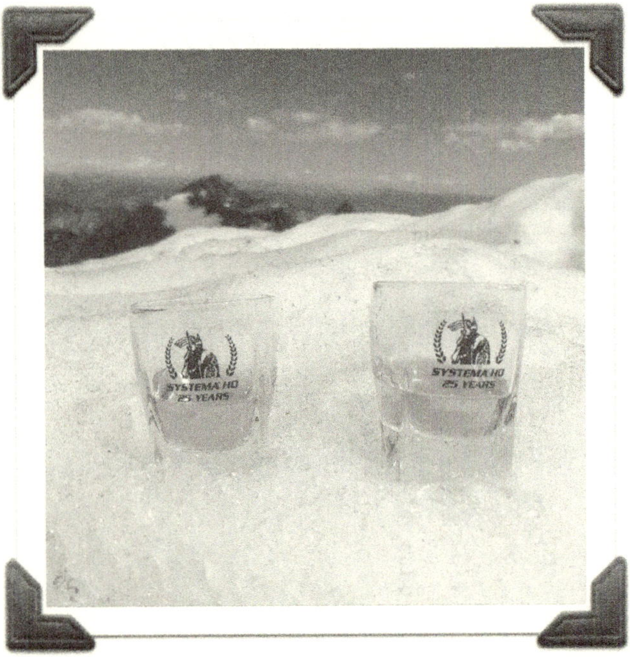
SYSTEMA HQ
25 YEARS
SYSTEMA HQ
25 YEARS

A few years ago I wrote:

"I realize that as much as I'd like to be a rugged individualist who can walk into the wild alone, that's not quite who I am. My need for solitude is in terms of hours, not days; and balanced by a need for solid people who understand.
I long for a brother-band. Men who will gather and create a flexible network to support each other and push one another onward.
IRON SHARPENS IRON
BLOOD CALLS TO BLOOD."

As John Mosby writes in 'Forging the Hero': "focus on developing this nucleus, even if it's just two of you."

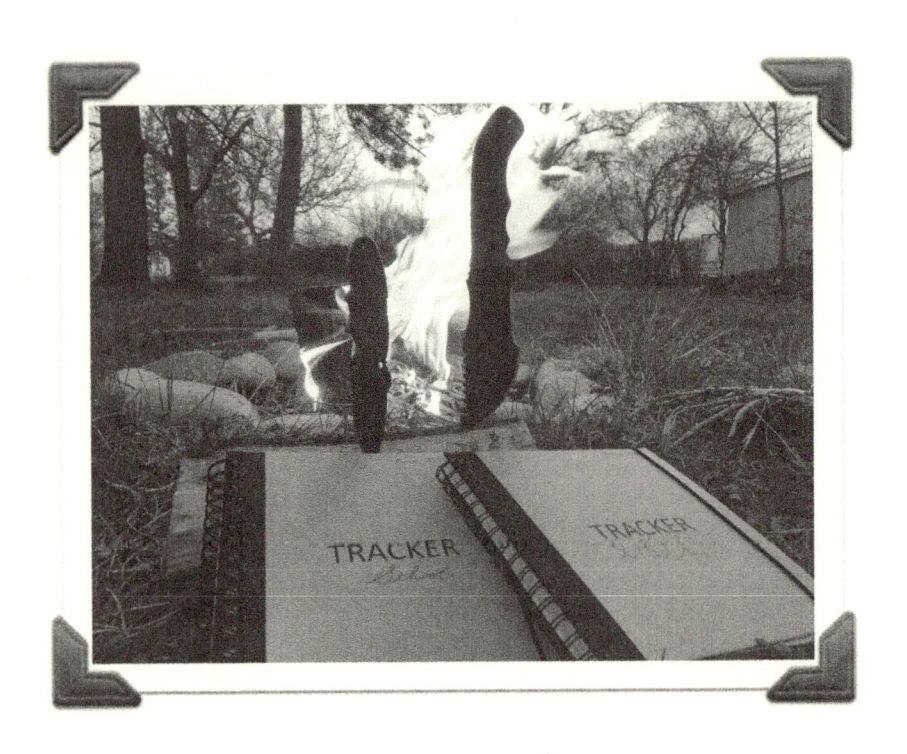

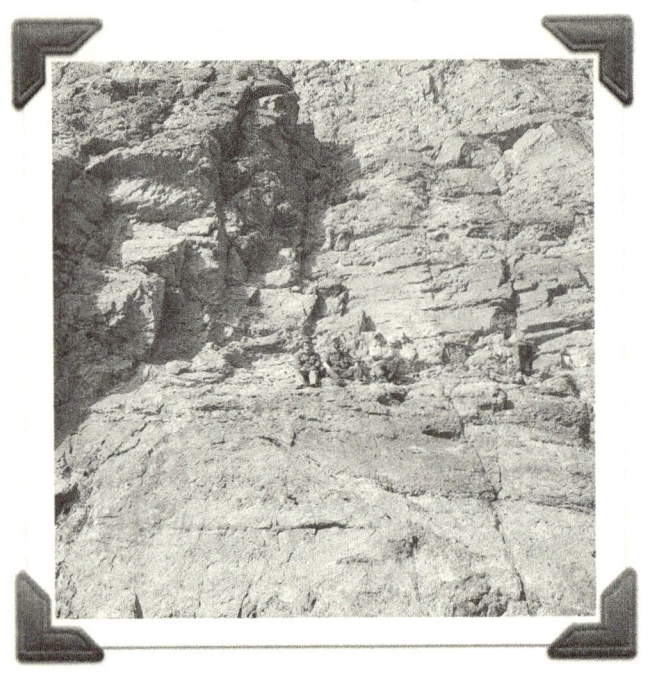

Practice list 2019:

- Marksmanship
- Weapons drills
- Archery
- Hand to hand combatives armed & unarmed
- First aid & trauma care
- Lockpicking
- Firebuilding
- Bird language & Awareness drills
- Physical conditioning
- Swimming
- Sailing
- Orienteering / land nav.
- Tracking
- Team movement
- Shelter

My vision for gatherings would include a sharp 30 to 45 min work out, time to work on any selected skill(s), cooking and eating, and potentially a movie if desired and time allows.

"Don't explain your philosophy.
Embody it."
– Epictetus

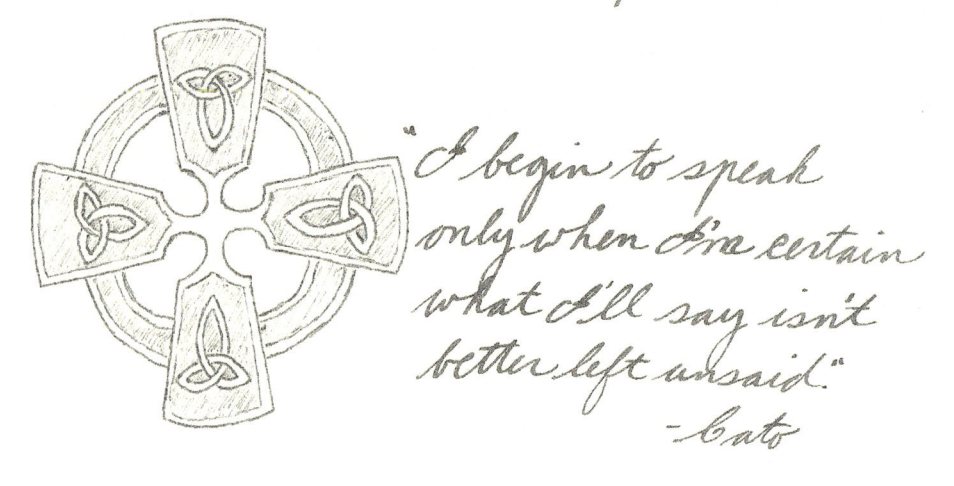

"I begin to speak
only when I'm certain
what I'll say isn't
better left unsaid."
– Cato

"The right word may be effective,
but no word was ever as effective
as a rightly timed pause."
– Mark Twain

"He who knows how to speak,
knows also when."
– Archimedes

"Men are like steel.
When they lose their temper,
they lose their worth."
- Anonymous

"You always own the option of having no opinion.
There is never any need to get worked up or to trouble your soul about things you can't control.
These things are not asking to be judged by you. Leave them alone."
— Marcus Aurelius

"A man may conquer a million men in battle but one who conquers himself is, indeed, the greatest of conquerors."
— Buddha

"Everything that irritates us about others,
can lead us to an understanding
        of ourselves."
                    - Carl Jung

"Our main business is not
to see what lies dimly
in the distance,
but to do what lies
clearly at hand."
        - Thomas Carlyle

If you focus on the hurt
you will continue to suffer.
If you focus on the lesson
you will continue to learn.
                - @kind.reminders

"Some days it's good to remind yourself...
"I am here to cross the swamp,
not to fight all the alligators."
            - Emmanuel Manolakakis

Deeper preparedness and local reliance

- buy food in bulk, store in food-grade plastic buckets.
    rice, beans, flour, raisins, nuts, seeds, oats, jars of oil, honey, vinegar
  Scale quantity to meet your need - 1 or 2 people might get 5 lb bags and store in a couple buckets; a family might consider 8 or 12 buckets and 50 lb quantities. Store buckets in a cool place if you can.

- store water - 1 gal. per person per day, minimum 3 days

- think about alternate heating and cooking sources
    SOLAR OVEN?
    WOOD STOVE?

- grow a garden, or help neighbors who garden
- build relationship with local farmers and producers
- preserve food - learn to can, get a dehydrator
  SOLAR DEHYDRATOR?
- work from home if you can cut commute time and cost, control your schedule.
- sensible precautions for the defense of your home and loved ones

BUY IT CHEAP, STACK IT DEEP. WHETHER "IT" IS A BAG OF RICE, A BOX OF SHOTSHELLS, OR A CASE OF TOILET PAPER, BUY AHEAD OF YOUR NEED.

Blind work

YOUR EYES CAN DECEIVE YOU,
    DON'T TRUST THEM.
STRETCH OUT WITH YOUR FEELINGS,
    YOU SEE? YOU CAN DO IT.
                    — OBI-WAN KENOBI
                    STAR WARS: A NEW HOPE

Blind work and intuition training go hand in hand.
When you work without sight, all other senses sharpen and kick into high gear.

Through both Tracker School and Systema, I've worked on exercises where a partner walks toward you from any direction, and you have to determine whether they are armed/threatening or neutral/friendly. Sometimes we see them, sometimes we close our eyes and sense them blind.

Stand and turn in a circle with your eyes shut for a minute, while your partner silently moves to 4 or 5 paces from you. Then point to the place you think he's standing and then open your eyes and see how accurate you were.

One year at Tracker School, we did a blindfolded drum stalk, affectionately known as 'blindfolds and bathing suits.' Though it was chilly, we stripped down to swim attire to increase sensory perception and put on blindfolds. Then we walked carefully towards the sound of a drum, struck a double beat every minute or two. The course was set through field and woods so we had to work around trees, bushes, and tents, and navigate undergrowth and variations in the terrain.

Another time at Tracker, we did quarter-staff forms while balanced on The Log, down over the swimming area. Everyone got wet that day. Later on we would practice on logs set on the ground around the main camp, and our balance was much better. Tom walked by and snorted, "What's changed? why's your balance so good up here, when it sucked down there? It's all in your head, gang."

One time I was teaching some blindfolded knife defense, slow motion thrusting or stabbing with dull metal training knives. I held my knife alongside my partner's abdomen with the edge down so there was no immediate threat. I could see the look of concentration on her face as she tried to figure it out.

Then I turned my wrist so the blade rotated 90°, and the cutting edge was poised an inch from her stomach. Immediately, her face changed to a look of discomfort and she took a step directly away from the trajectory of my blade.

At Camp 2018, one evening in the dark, Vladimir pulled me to demo this. I had my eyes closed while he had the knife. Every time I felt a pressure approaching part of my body, I would move that area away. Vlad said, "Oh! He's quite good! I don't know if you can see, but I can."

Later, working with a training partner, I felt my knees loosen so I dropped low, and he said "Hey! Are your eyes open? You just completely ducked under a slash toward your head!"

Another year, Vlad suggested that anyone interested should train for an entire afternoon blindfolded.

I blindfolded early and sat on a rock for 30 minutes listening and feeling. Then I asked my friend Dean to guide me along the quarter-mile trail to the training area in the woods. He said "Okay, let's run!"

I grabbed his shoulder and we were off.

We trained all afternoon, full combative practice. Different, without sight.

On the way back in, there's a fallen log partly overhanging the trail; Dean is a bit shorter than me and ran right under it. Then there was a resounding "thunk!" as my forehead ran into it and a gasp from other students, and Dean said "Don't worry! He's fine!"

And on we ran!

I was relaxed from the afternoon practice and the breath training we do to release the shock of impact, and I was fine.

We kept going to do fighting in the water, and I kept my blindfold.

Next camp, I returned the favor by guiding him into a clothesline full of towels.

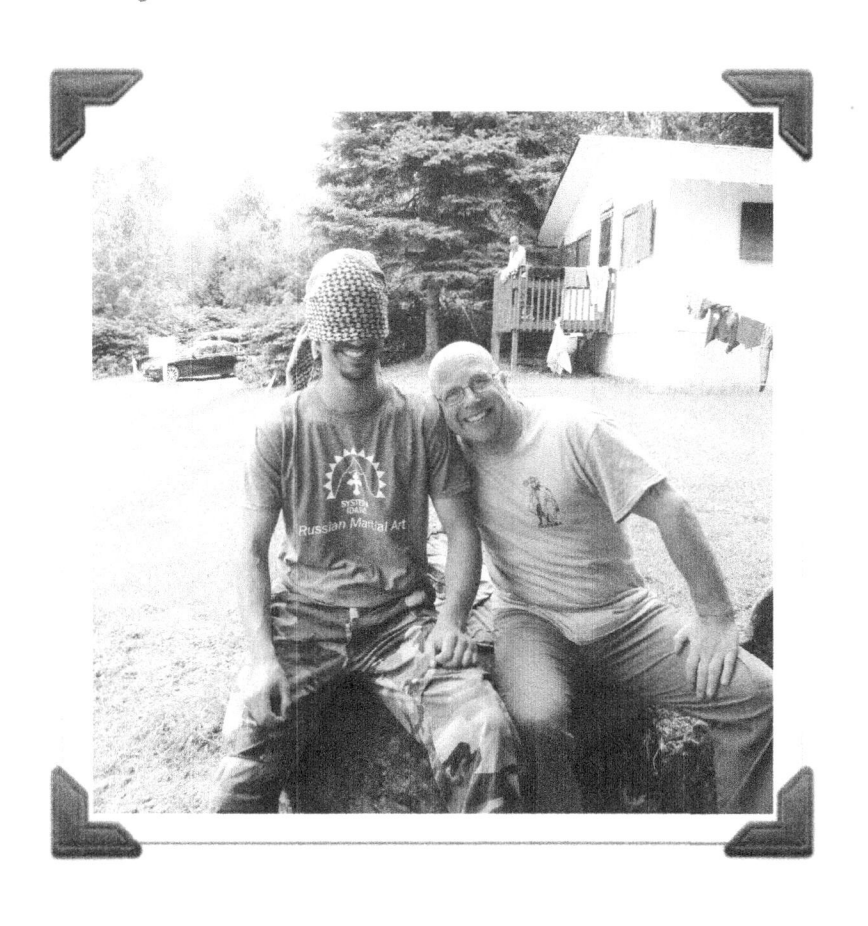

Short Swords
by ArtofManliness.com

Oliver Wendell Holmes once wrote that a people "that shortens its weapons lengthens its boundaries."

By this he meant that men who were capable of fighting at close quarters also possessed the essential courage, the 'thumos', that ultimately won battles, turned the tide of war — protected and expanded the boundaries of their nation. Spartan warriors, for example, carried swords just a foot long, which they thrust into an enemy's throat or groin when the space between the battle lines grew so thin that their spears were no longer effective.

In contrast, troops that relied on weapons that put greater distance between the combatant and his foe — lances carried on horseback, javelins hurled from a place of safety, arrows shot from on high — lacked the requisite 'andreia', the manliness, that would win out in the end.

Holmes didn't mean his epigram literally, in that longer-range weapons never offer strategic advantage. Rather, he was making the point that the men who can back up their technology with the bravery to fight hand-to-hand are those who come out on top.

This principle truly applies beyond the battlefield to every area of life. Especially in a time when it's easy to attempt to execute one's strategy from behind the safety of technological screens, success goes to the man who's still able to step right up to the threshold of risk, conflict and challenge — who can talk to people face-to-face, have difficult conversations in person, ask directly for what he wants, put himself out there. The man who ceases to do endless research and finally takes action; who feels the hot breath of opposition when he grasps the barbell, approaches a woman, steps up to a podium; is he who gains the victory, expands his empire, lengthens his boundaries.

Physical training is a bare minimum. It doesn't make you a warrior, or a savage, or a beast, or some kind of mythical mixture of lion, viking, and wolf.

It means you have placed a hand on the lowest and simplest rung on the ladder that leads to both self-transformation and self-maintenance, and there's a long way to go, yet.

This being said, because of it's foundational nature, it is also one of the most important things to begin and continue on the road of Total Life Reform.

Lots of good things are like that:
  simple, fundamental, critical.

Just don't pretend it makes you the Übermensch because you've picked up a barbell — there are enough assholes in the world already.

— Paul Waggener
Operation Werewolf

Nowadays, fear is big currency.

+ Everywhere you go, everywhere you look, big media and industry titans spread the fear of "not enough."

+ The fear of war, sickness, recession, violence, poverty, or being singled out for holding on to unpopular truths.

+ It's bullshit.

+ Don't buy stock in their currency — it doesn't have a future.

+ What does have a future is setting down the phone, turning off the news, and investing time with your peer group creating lasting things of value that matter.

+ That's a currency they can't devalue.

+ Stop bringing fear into the village.

+ #operationwerewolf

KEEP FEAR TO YOURSELF —
SHARE COURAGE WITH OTHERS

BOOKS

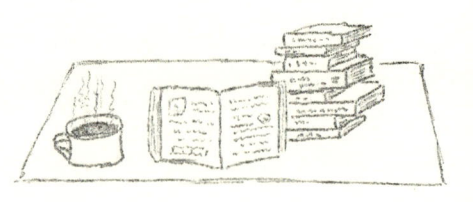

STRENGTH:

- CONVICT CONDITIONING — Wade
- CONVICT CONDITIONING 2 — Wade
- SIMPLE & SINISTER — Pavel
- THE QUICK AND THE DEAD — Pavel
- RAISING THE BAR — Kavadlo
- PUSHING THE LIMITS — Kavadlo
- COMBAT STRENGTH TRAINING — McNamara
- PARKOUR AND FREERUNNING HANDBOOK — Edwardes

AWARENESS:

- WHAT THE ROBIN KNOWS — Young
- LEFT OF BANG — Van Horne
- NATURE OBSERVATION AND TRACKING — Brown
- TACTICAL TRACKING OPERATIONS — Scott-Donelan

TOP 3:

- NATURAL BORN HEROES — McDougall
- LET EVERY BREATH... — Vasiliev
- ONE SECOND AFTER — Forstchen

MARTIAL ARTS:

- STRIKES: SOUL MEETS BODY — Vasiliev
- EDGE: SECRETS OF THE RUSSIAN BLADEMASTERS — Vasiliev
- THE RUSSIAN SYSTEM GUIDEBOOK — Vasiliev
- SYSTEMA MANUAL — Komarov
- THE SYSTEMA WARRIOR GUIDEBOOK — Mayberry
- KODOKAN JUDO — Kano
- MIND OVER MUSCLE — Kano
- HIGHER JUDO — Feldenkrais
- VITAL JUDO — Sato & Okano
- JIU-JITSU UNIVERSITY — Ribeiro
- WHEN VIOLENCE IS THE ANSWER — Larkin

SURVIVAL:

WILDERNESS SURVIVAL - Brown
100 DEADLY SKILLS - Emerson
100 DEADLY SKILLS: SURVIVAL EDITION - Emerson
SENTINEL - McNamara
PROTECTING OTHERS - Wagner
THE DARK SECRETS OF SHTF SURVIVAL - Begovic
WHERE THERE IS NO DOCTOR - Werner

HEALTH:

NOURISHING TRADITIONS - Fallon
HOW TO EAT, MOVE AND BE HEALTHY - Chek
HIDDEN MESSAGES IN WATER - Emoto

FORAGING:

WILD EDIBLE AND MEDICINAL PLANTS - Brown
WILD WISDOM OF WEEDS - Blair
DANDELION HUNTER - Lerner

MOTIVATION:

12 RULES FOR LIFE - Peterson
DISCIPLINE EQUALS FREEDOM - Willink
THE WARRIOR ETHOS - Pressfield

"You will never be alone with a poet in your pocket." - John Adams

TRIBE:

FORGING THE HERO - Mosby
THE WAY OF MEN - Donovan
BECOMING A BARBARIAN - Donovan
SOVEREIGNTY - Michler
WILD AT HEART - Eldredge

TACTICAL:

RELUCTANT PARTISAN 1 & 2 - Mosby
GUERRILLA GUNFIGHTER - Mosby
THE TIGERS WAY - Poole
RATTENKRIEG - Taubert
FRY THE BRAIN - West

INSPIRATION:

- THE WAY OF THE SCOUT — Brown
- ANGELS IN IRON — Prata
- THE WARWOLF — Lins
- GATES OF FIRE — Pressfield
- EXODUS — Uris
- MILA 18 — Uris
- MY SIDE OF THE MOUNTAIN — George
- THE FAR SIDE OF THE MOUNTAIN — George
- ROGUE HEROES — MacIntyre
- SCHOOL OF THE MOON — McHardy
- FAIR BLOWS THE WIND — L'Amour
- THE WALKING DRUM — L'Amour
- CAPTAIN BLOOD — Sabatini
- NARNIA* — Lewis
- ANYTHING BY TOLKIEN*
- SHERLOCK HOLMES* — Doyle
- LORD PETER WIMSEY* — Sayers
- THE DOLPHIN CYCLE* — Sutcliff
- JAMES BOND* — Fleming
- THE TRACKER — Brown
- THE SEARCH — Brown
- GRANDFATHER — Brown
- CASE FILES OF THE TRACKER — Brown
- GERONIMO — w/ Barrett
- WATCH FOR ME ON THE MOUNTAIN — Carter
- EMPIRE OF THE SUMMER MOON — Gwynne
- ANOTHER MANS WAR — Childers
- THE DEVILS GUARD — Elford
- THE EAGLE HAS LANDED — Higgins
- ON WINGS OF EAGLES — Follet
- 13 HOURS — Zuckoff
- KILLING ROMMEL — Pressfield
- INTO THE LIONS MOUTH — Loftis
- THE GIFT OF RAIN — Eng
- GARDEN OF THE EVENING MISTS — Eng
- LAYS OF ANCIENT ROME — Macaulay
- FATHER BROWN OMNIBUS — Chesterton
- THE BALLAD OF THE WHITE HORSE — Chesterton
- THE MAN WHO WAS THURSDAY — Chesterton
- THE FOUNDATION — Asimov
- THE REVENGE OF THE SITH — Stover
- THE THREE MUSKETEERS — Dumas
- THE COUNT OF MONTE CRISTO — Dumas

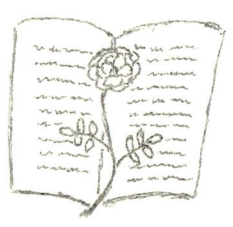

* series

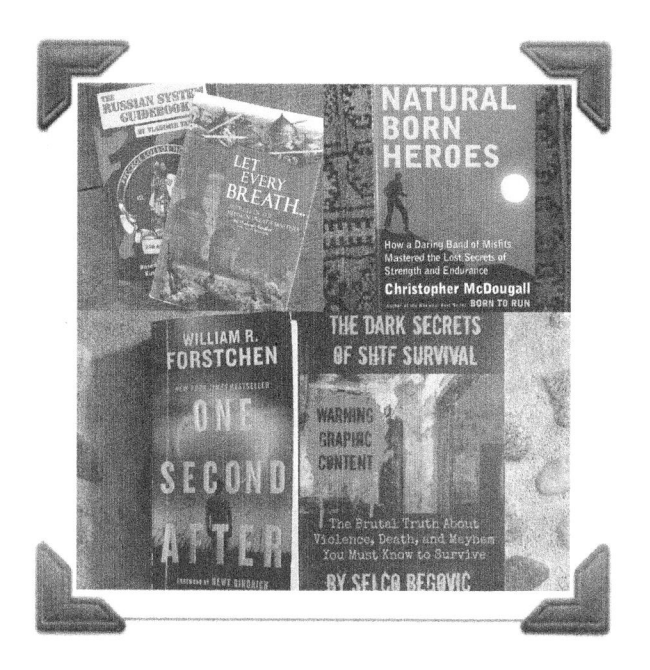

Good reading is always welcome, these are a few of my favorites that show up prominently on the reading list in Share the Gift.

Let Every Breath.... and The Russian System Guidebook both have valuable advice for breathwork and exercise to release stress and tension and build up your health and immune system.

Natural Born Heroes has a variety of info on most of my favorite subjects. Good read!

One Second After is a good novel that walks through a collapse from an EMP strike, in a fairly realistic manner. Good story and brings up questions or thought provoking info.

Dark Secrets is by a guy who lived through the Balkan War in the '90s, and shares his experience. Most helpful takeaway: do not panic! Watch carefully, prepare yourself, and do not let the media stampede you into a panic with the rest of the herd.

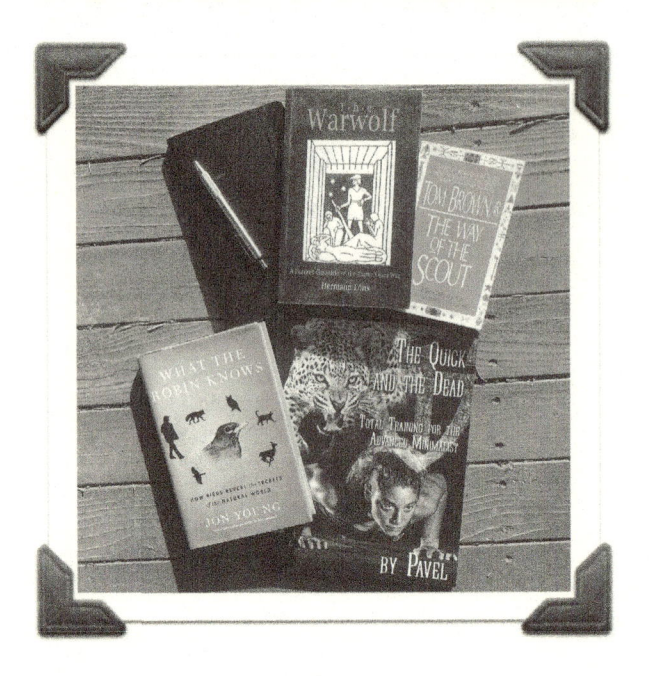

The Way of the Scout, the book that got me started on the Tracker School path. Lots of adventures from Tom Brown Jr's training.

The Warwolf, written before the First World War about German farmers during the Thirty Years War (1618-1648) who had to move deep into the moors, rebuild fortified settlements, and organize networks of scouts and roving patrols to defend against the ill disciplined soldiery of all sides in that conflict. Good book!

The Quick and the Dead, one of my favorite kettlebell workout regimes, built by StrongFirst to fit in a busy schedule and promote health and endurance by training your mitochondria to oxygenate more efficiently. Fascinating science and a straightforward program.

What the Robin Knows, bird language, concentric rings, and how to read them. Well written and accessible, this study opens wide dimensions into the natural world.

Journal, take some notes, let off some steam, document your observations and experiences. How does stress affect you and the people around you? I think the corona virus is a warmup round, and look at how quickly the panic took hold! What can you do to put yourself on a better footing for the next crisis?

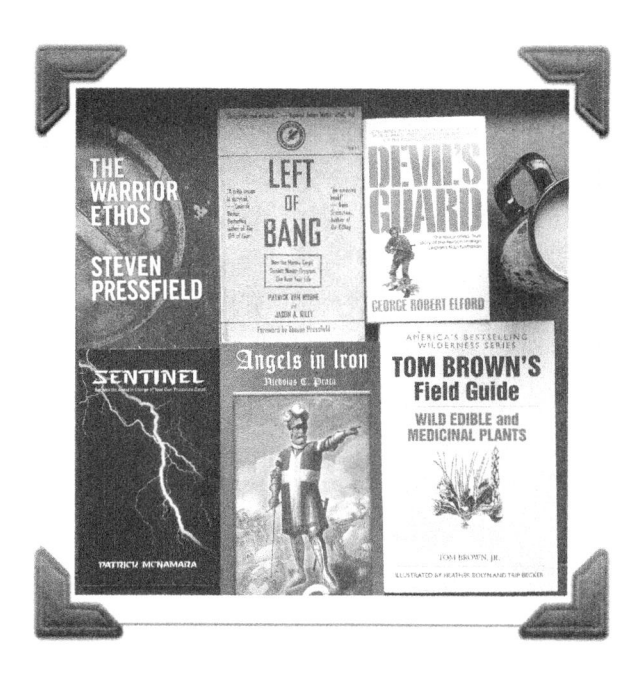

Angels in Iron, about the first siege of Malta in 1565. One of my favorite stories of siege and seems fitting as many people are quarantined inside; at least we're not worried about cannon fire against our walls!
Cannon fire and knights in battle on the walls and in the trenches, knives in the water and the tunnels.

Wild Edible and Medicinal Plants, I like this guide book because Tom goes through 100 plants not just giving descriptions, properties, uses, and preparation for each plant, but also a short story of how he learned each one. The stories help me remember the information, and it's fun reading.

Sentinel, prepare yourself to take care of you and yours. Be your own bodyguard. Follow Patrick McNamara @tmacsinc for more quality info!

Warrior Ethos, Steven Pressfield delves into the mentality and spirit of the warrior. Short book, good thoughts.

Left of Bang, the study of awareness and how people move and interact and what we can learn from some very basic and universal cues. Fascinating study!

Devil's Guard, the story of SS troopers joining the French Foreign Legion after WW2 and going on to fight in French Vietnam. There's some debate about whether this is a true story, but I could see it happening, and the Foreign Legion covering it for pr reasons. In any case it's a well written narrative and showcases some interesting tactics.

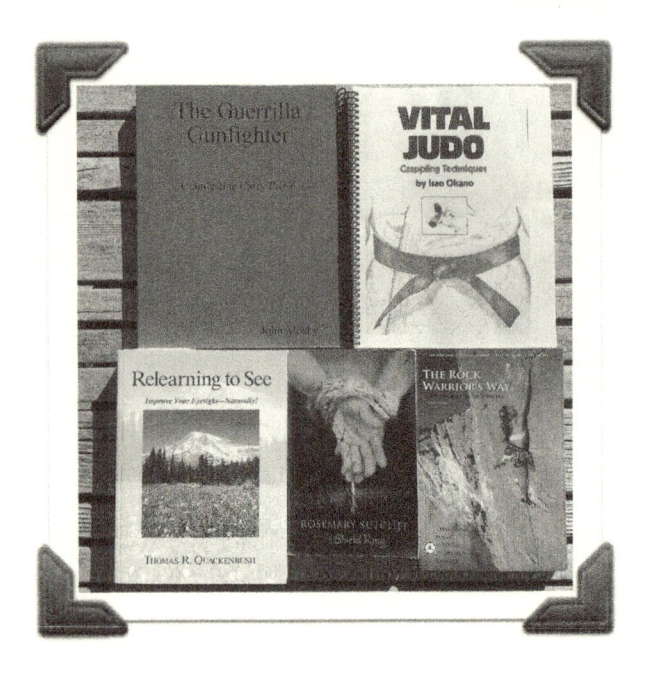

Keep the mind alive and the body will follow.

The Rock Warriors Way, mental training for rock climbing, and life, drawing heavily on the warrior tradition. Looks helpful for anyone wanting to work on themselves, hone their focus, and reduce or eliminate the influence of the Ego.

The Shield Ring, the last volume of the Dolphin Cycle. This is one of my favorite series of historical fiction, it starts in the First Century with the search for the Lost Ninth Legion, continues up through the Roman withdrawal from Britain and the Saxon invasions, has an excellent historical rendition of Arthur, and then this book which I recently learned about, finishes the series well after the Norman Invasion when they finally conquer the last Norse/Saxon stronghold in the Lake District.

Vital Judo: Grappling Techniques, one of my Judo Sensei's recommended this and its companion volume of throwing techniques, but said they were long out of print. Fortunately you can dig around online and find pdf's for a few dollars or even for free. And the local copy shop will print it out and bind it. Great material!

Guerrilla Gunfighter: Clandestine Carry Pistol, good material for anyone thinking about regular concealed carry. Drills, training procedures, how to set up your training, why to carry, this guy is good. A bit salty, but I like his style.

Relearning to See, many sight issues stem from tension or imbalance in the muscles that control the eye. If you retrain those muscles to the proper levels of tension working together, then sight improves.

I wear glasses to drive since my sight is just below the legal requirement. But I dislike wearing lenses for the rest of my active life. A good friend recommended this book years ago, and I've done some of the exercises here and there, now is a good time for me to focus on it and *see* what I can do.

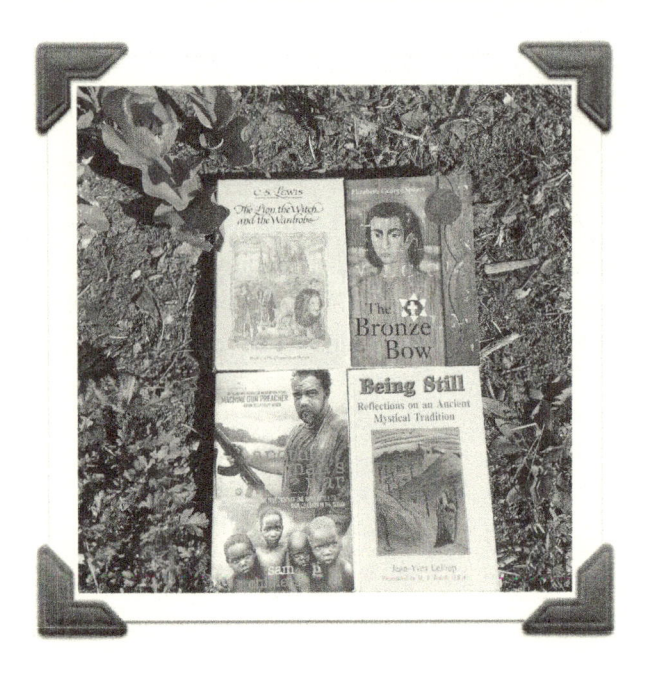

The Lion the Witch and the Wardrobe; excellent children's fantasy, with battle, betrayal, redemption, and one of the best allegories of the resurrection. This is a classic that's just as enjoyable for adults as for children.
My dad started reading Narnia to me when I was two or three years old, probably a large part of the reason I grew up with a sword in my hand. We would read the whole series aloud as a family every year for most of my growing up.

The Bronze Bow; historical fiction about a young Zealot in the first century, and his meeting with the Christ. Lots of action, but also makes you pause and ponder.

Another Mans War; there in no greater love than to lay down your life for another. Sam Childers was a motorcycle gangster and drug dealer before God turned his life around, then he put his skill in violence to helping the orphans in South Sudan, rescuing kids from the bush when no one else would risk confronting the rebel armies of Joseph Kony. Good book, and the movie is pretty good too.

Being Still; an introduction to the Hesychistic practice of meditation and prayer, and a comparison to other major religious disciplines around the world. Beautiful.

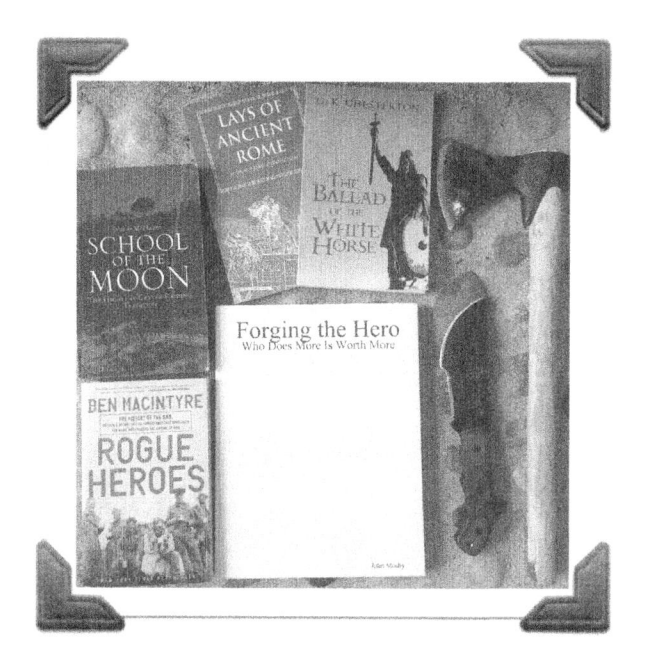

Forging the Hero, starts off with a nice history of the trends of failing empires, and then launches into a lengthy treatise on building resilient clan and tribe to weather that storm. So far I really like everything I've read by John Mosby, Mountain Guerrilla.

Rogue Heroes, classic history of the British SAS from their foundation in the North African desert through Italy and France to the end of WWII. I like modern special ops stories, but I really like the older ones when they were up against a technologically superior foe and ingenuity and bold tactics had to carry the day.

School of the Moon, who doesn't like a little Scottish highland raiding? Out of print but worth the read if you track down a copy.

The Ballad of the White Horse, and The Lays of Ancient Rome, two of my favorite works of poetry. Especially Horatius at the Bridge in the Lays, and the battles at Ethandune in the Ballad.

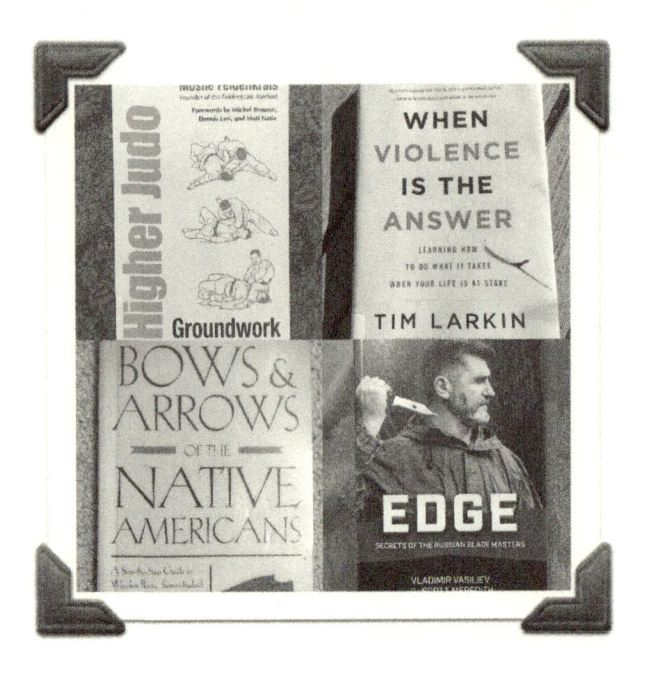

When Violence is the Answer is fascinating with its research into violent encounters, who perpetuates then, and how to build build awareness and skills to survive and/or avoid. Very well done!

Higher Judo, written by a physicist in the 30s, great scientific approach to the philosophy of judo, and the mechanics of newaza or fighting on the ground; and this guy worked with the Haganah in Israel and had combat experience to work with too.

Edge: Secrets of the Russian Bkademasters, Vlad's latest book, dealing with knifework and including solo and partner training. Vlad's books are all great!

Bows & Arrows of the Native Americans, good read on building your own archery equipment. I haven't taken the steps to build my own yet, but it's still a goal!

Read, learn, practice, enjoy!

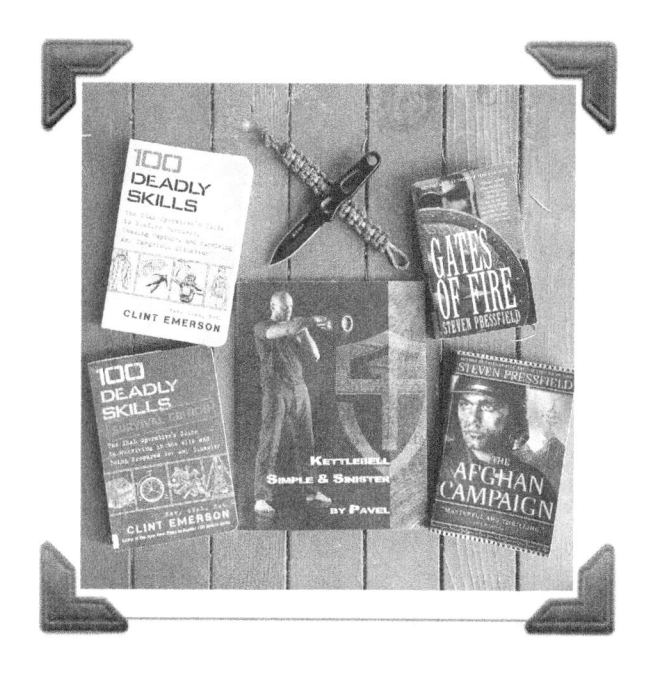

Kettlebell: Simple & Sinister by Strongfirst, my favorite kettlebell program, and my go-to recommendation whenever anyone asks me for kettlebell training advice.

100 Deadly Skills, both books are packed with valuable info. Each skill is given a couple pages including illustrations in a graphic novel style and a more detailed write-up. Good stuff in an accessible and entertaining format. And I just heard there's a third book in the works! 100 Deadly Skills has been an influence and inspiration in my writing. Thank you sir!

The Gates of Fire, the story of the Spartans at Thermopylae. One of my favorite books. Beautiful, gripping, intense, brutal. Ancient warfare and the timeless loyalty of soldiers to one another.

The Afghan Campaign, Alexander the Great in Afghanistan. It's striking to see similarities between the war in the middle-East in 300BC and current wars in those mountains. Some things don't change, regardless the weapons and technology, the people who live or fight there are incredibly tough.

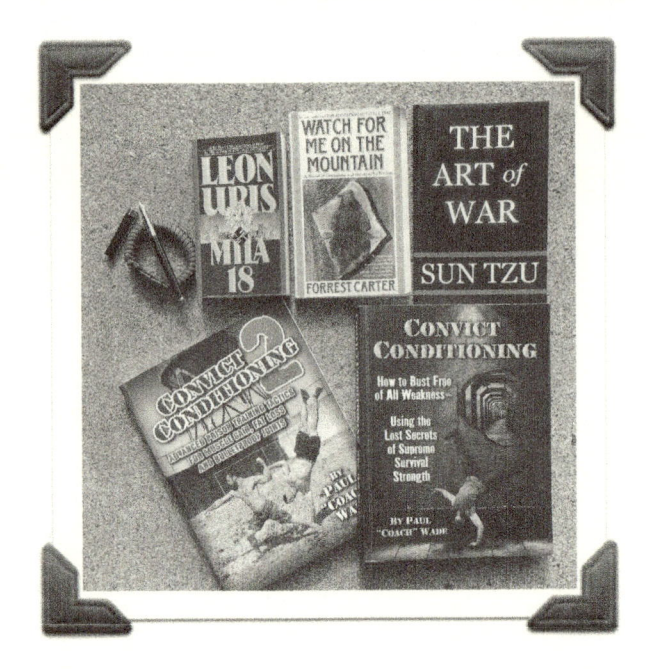

Convict Conditioning and CC2 are great books for calisthenics progressions. I've used this program a lot. The Big Six exercises are thoughtfully laid out with 10 steps that progress from easy moves anyone can start with, up to elite feats like pistol squats and one arm pull-ups. Simple strength training, but not easy!

Mila 18, Leon Uris' epic novel of the Jewish Ghetto in Warsaw during the war. ordinary people turned resistance fighters held off SS units for a month, with only small arms and bricks.

Watch For Me On The Mountain, the life of Geronimo. Historical fiction, but so good! To shelter ones people and guide them to safety, and sacrifice to protect them.

The Art of War, the oldest known book of tactical wisdom. Enough said.

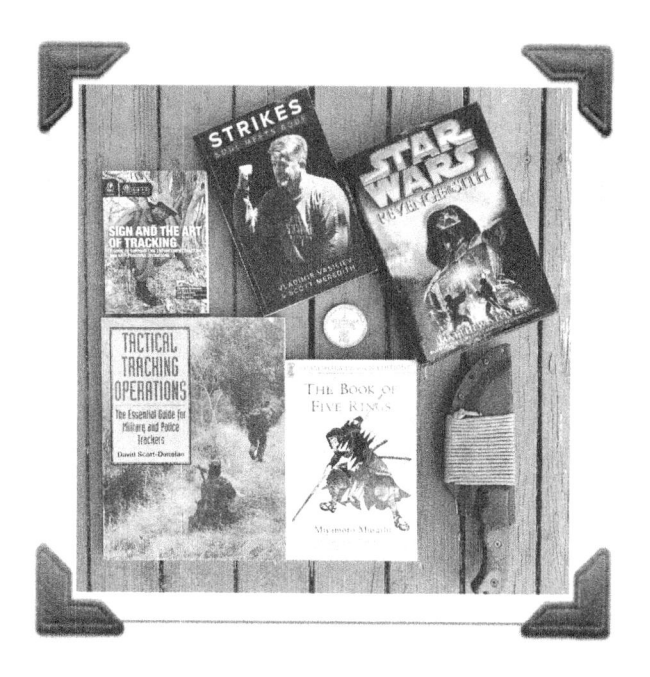

Tactical Tracking Operations, a different school and a complimentary approach to the Tracker School classes I've taken. David Scott-Donelan served in the Rhodesian SAS and RLI, and his info is fantastic: tracking, gear, weapons, and a smattering of stories. I haven't had a chance to train with him yet, but I know people who have and highly recommend it. This book is out of print now, but if you find a copy, snatch it!

Sign and the Art of Tracking, another book I got from David Scott-Donelan. Good information on tracking basics, land nav, gear, and diet. "The perception of a lightly clad Native American or San Bushman tracker with knife and shoulder bag, fire kit and bow is a good ideal."

The Book of Five Rings, classic wisdom from one of the foremost swordsman of the human race.

Strikes: Soul Meets Body, my teacher's book on the Systema methodology of delivering and receiving strikes, and much more. Worth rereading every year!

Star Wars: Revenge of the Sith, where the movie was lacking, the novel delivers! I loved this book as a teenager, and picking it up again recently, it's just as good as I remember. Matthew Stover brilliantly captures the drama of galaxy at war and the emotion of the descent into darkness. One of my favorites!

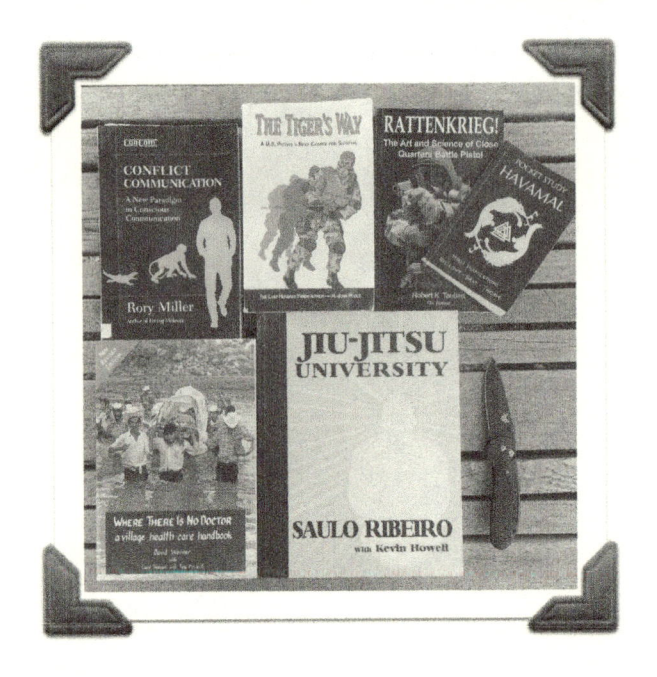

Conflict Communication is my current read, and quickly becoming a favorite. Thoughtfully written, this is quite a resource for improving communication both in stressful environments and in everyday life.

The Tigers Way, a fascinating exploration of Eastern Tactics from a variety of wars in the last century and how to apply those lessons.

Rattenkrieg, pistol combat techniques as taught by an FBI instructor. Solid resource.

Where There Is No Doctor, this book was written for healthcare workers in remote areas of the world. Lots to be learned here. I believe it is available as a pdf for free download, but I bought the book because paperbacks don't need batteries.

Jiu-Jitsu University, step by step manual of grappling technique illustrated with color photos on every page, including lots of photos of both correct technique and common errors to avoid. Excellent!

The Havamal, wisdom of the Ancient North. Ostensibly the sayings of Odin, King of the Aesir, but some good advice in any case.

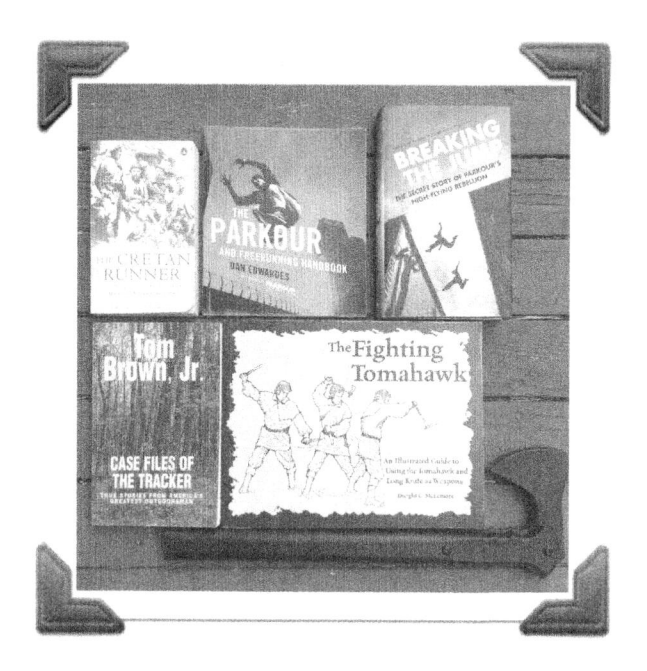

The Fighting Tomahawk, a how-to manual to study this devastating weapon of the American past.
Illustrated with lots of pen and ink drawing, this was one of the first books I started copying illustrations from for my training journal, and helped me realize how much more I enjoy notes when I put pictures with them.

The Parkour and Freerunning Handbook, great start into the world of parkour. Guidance for safety and efficiency, training ideas, and some pretty cool inspiration.

Breaking the Jump, the underground history of parkour, really cool read!

The Cretan Runner, stories from one of the best Resistance fighters from the Isle of Crete. Known for his endurance and audacity, he could run for miles through mountain ranges of broken rock carrying messages, and turn right around to run back a reply.

The Case Files of The Tracker, more stories of Tom Brown, tracking people and animals. Most notably a soldier he trained who went rogue; that was the story The Hunted was based on. Good story, good movie.

"Like Odin and Thor,
we know we will die,
but unless we fight, we're
already as good as dead.
Better to live vigorously,
better to fight, than simply
wait for the end... in peace."
— Becoming a Barbarian

"Death smiles at us all,
all a man can do
is smile back."
— Marcus Aurelius

"When your time comes to die
be not like those whose
hearts are filled with fear of death.
So that when their time comes
they weep and pray for a little
more time to live their lives
over again in a different way.
Sing your death song
and die
like a hero going home."
— Tecumseh

The Prayer of the Optina Elders

O Lord, grant me with tranquility of soul to meet all that the coming day may bring. Grant me to surrender myself completely to Thy holy will. At every hour of this day guide and sustain me in all things. Whatsoever tidings I may receive in the course of the day, teach me to receive them with peace of soul and the firm conviction that all is in Thy holy will. Govern Thou my thoughts and feelings in all my words and deeds. In all unforeseen circumstances let me not forget that all cometh down from Thee. Teach me to deal uprightly and prudently with every member of my family, disturbing and grieving none.

O Lord, grant me strength to bear the weariness of the coming day and all events in the course of the day. Govern Thou my will and teach me to pray, to believe, to hope, to be patient, to forgive, and to love. Amen.

Peace is elusive.
If it exists at all when you search for it.
Shattered pieces, scattered on the wind.
I read once an old Orthodox saint
who wrote that "in pursuing peace,
many have lost it."

So lift the war hammer high,
as thunder booms and roars
and lightning slashes
across the sky.
Christ Himself said, "I come
not to bring peace, but a sword."
Take up the battle sword, and ride!

I seek no longer for peace,
but to take the adventure that comes.
And in not seeking peace,
moments of serenity find me more often.
I stand still in the shadow of
the Cross. I will walk through many
doors, and worship with many people.
But my heart yearns for the
mountains and the free air,
God's country.

"The only thing necessary for the triumph of evil is that good men should do nothing."
— Edmund Burke

"Become what evil fears."
— Joe Mayberry

Made in the USA
Monee, IL
12 May 2021